Surgery of the Liver and Portal Circulation

SURGERY OF THE LIVER AND PORTAL CIRCULATION

William V. McDermott, Jr., M. D.

David W. and David Cheever Professor of Surgery, Harvard Medical School. Director, Harvard Surgical Service (New England Deaconess, Cambridge, Faulkner and Mount Auburn Hospitals). Director, Sears Surgical Laboratories, Boston City Hospital. Director, Cancer Research Institute, New England Deaconess Hospital

LEA & FEBIGER · 1974 · PHILADELPHIA

Library of Congress Cataloging in Publication Data

McDermott, William V 1917—
Surgery of the liver and portal circulation.

1. Liver—Surgery. 2. Portal hypertension.
I. Title. [DNLM: 1. Liver—Surgery. 2. Liver circulation.
3. Liver diseases—Pathology. WJ700 M134s 1974]
RD546.M18 1974 617'.556 73-12569

ISBN 0-8121-0393-9

Library of Congress Catalog Card Number 73-12569

Published in Great Britain by Henry Kimpton Publishers, London

PRINTED IN THE UNITED STATES OF AMERICA

To the memory of Blanche
and
To my wife, Jane

Preface

This volume, unlike texts of multiple authorship, is intended to present the views of one individual on the complex pathophysiology of diseases of the liver and portal circulation, and the problems inherent in their surgical treatment.

The inadequacies of single authorship are obvious. Spirited controversy exists in almost all areas of pathophysiology; innumerable ingenious and satisfactory operative techniques have been developed which differ from those presented in this volume; and many experienced surgeons would disagree with proposed methods of evaluation and management. On the other hand, a series of chapters, each written by an expert, invariably results in some duplications and omissions and tends to lack continuity of thought. The ultimate objective of this volume is to provide the general surgeon with a simplified guide to management from a single point of view.

Consistent with this particular approach, the text has not been documented with endless references, but the bibliography given at the end of each chapter is intended to provide the reader with a list of valuable monographs and specific reports concerned with each particular section. The bibliography is not intended to be totally comprehensive and many excellent, provocative, and important references may be missing. If, however, the reader wishes to explore in depth any of these areas, more specific details and references can be found in the bibliography of listed texts, monographs, and reports. With the text serving as an introduction, the reader may pursue almost endlessly a chain of historical thought and current controversy, using the listed bibliography as a base.

In many sections, particularly those pertaining to surgical anatomy, and to biochemistry and pathophysiology of the liver, the text and illustrations have been kept to a minimum in the interest of avoiding a repetition of material easily available in standard, widely utilized textbooks. It is hoped that this brevity will prove advantageous to some and will not seriously offend others who might wish for a more expanded, extensive, and documented review of all topics presented.

I would like to express my appreciation to my surgical and medical colleagues throughout the country whose clinical and laboratory investigations have done so much to clarify the problems in this area, to faculty and research fellows at the Harvard Medical School whose association over the years has been so stimulating, and to the students whose provocative questions have been the stimulus for so many of the investigations described. Miss Zelda Cushner is responsible not only for the completion and accuracy of the manuscript but has provided constant suggestions and criticisms which have served to improve immeasurably the initial effort. Jayne McGuire, Barbara Kern, and Marguerite Souza have, as always, been continuously helpful with the endless details concerned with the final text. Dr. Melvin Clouse and Dr. Herbert Gramm of the Department of Radiology at the New England Deaconess Hospital were most helpful in the preparation of the chapter on Diagnostic Techniques in Liver Surgery.

William V. McDermott, Jr.

Boston, Massachusetts

Contents

Anatomy of the Liver and Portal Bed

CHAPTER 1

Excellent descriptions of the comparative anatomy and embryology of the liver can be found in a standard text of anatomy and embryology and in a number of existing books on the liver, particularly those of Child, Schiff and Schwartz. The details of the basic gross and microscopic anatomy are also easily available. Therefore, a detailed review of these areas would seem repetitious and unnecessary; only selected material and information that may be particularly pertinent to the problems encountered by the surgeon will be included in this chapter.

The embryologic development of the liver begins in about the fourth week in the life of the fetus when the hepatic diverticulum arises from the intradermal lining of the foregut. The tubular hepatic cords penetrate the septum transversum. Lobules develop, proliferating parenchymal cells become transformed into sinusoids, bile ductules form as centers of small parenchymal masses and ultimately the final form of the liver and its vascular and secretory apparatus takes place.

From the fifth to the seventh week of fetal development, a number of interesting changes take place in the blood flow to the fetal liver. The right omphalomesenteric vein becomes obliterated, and the left persists, developing ultimately into the main portal vein. The main flow of the umbilical vein becomes encompassed by the developing liver and shifts from the sinus venosus to the intrahepatic pathway, which becomes known as the ductus venosus. The ductus exists up to the birth of the fetus, providing a mechanism whereby oxygenated blood is carried directly to the heart; at birth, because of physiologic changes induced by respiration and a lowering of umbilical vein pressure, the ductus venosus closes off. Normally it closes off entirely, an interesting protective mechanism, which prevents any severe hemorrhage from the umbilical cord. This obliterated umbilical vein persists in the round ligament and provides a potential mechanism for access to the portal circulation that has been exploited for diagnostic and sometimes therapeutic purposes in recent years. As will be pointed out later, this obliterated vein can usually be identified and dilated and passage into the left portal vein achieved through gentle pressure on the dilator, which breaks through the thin septum occluding the hepatic end of the vein.

topographic anatomy

The segmental anatomy of the liver has been reasonably well defined and is shown in Figure 1-1. In contrast to that of the lung, however, the segmental anatomy of the liver is relatively unimportant to the surgeon since the types of segmental resections that can be carried out so well in the lung are not possible in the liver because of the interlocking and traversing pattern of the inflow and outflow from the hepatic artery and portal vein and the outflow from the

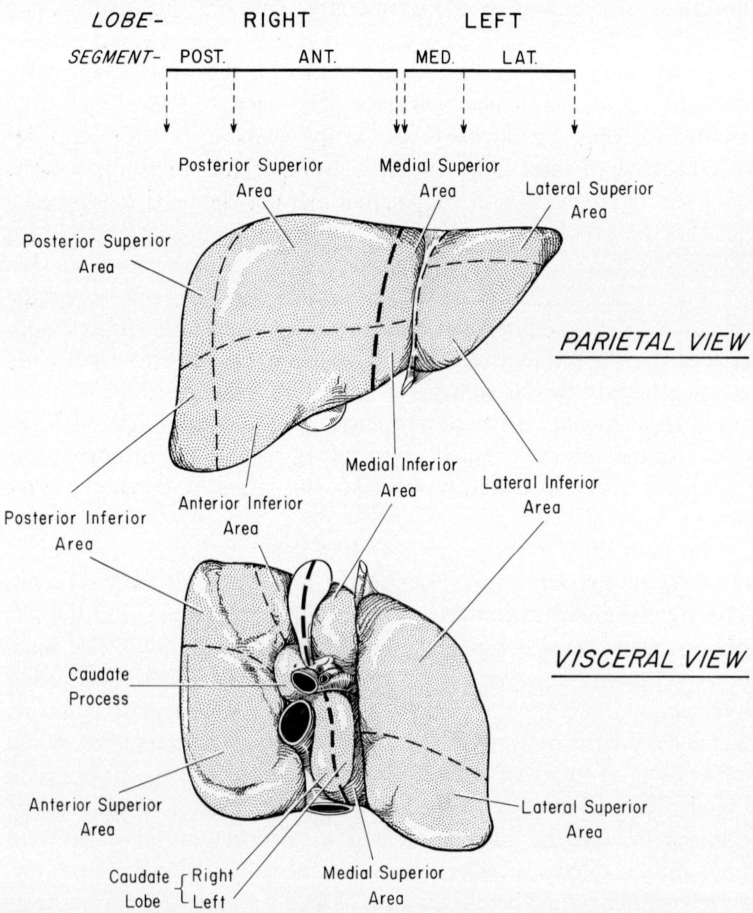

FIG. 1-1. Segmental anatomy of the liver

sinusoids and central and hepatic veins. In terms of surgical resection, one is usually limited to wedge resections, which are defined only as technical possibilities related to the thickness and configuration of the liver, and to major resections of the right and left lobes. In terms of specific localization of intrahepatic tumors, abscesses or cysts, and for more exact surgical descriptions, the segments as shown may be useful. The techniques of anatomic hepatic resection will be described in more detail, but in terms of gross anatomy and vascular supply, ligation of the right branches of the hepatic artery and portal vein will result in a line of demarcation between the major right and left lobes appearing 2 to 4 cm. lateral to the attachment of the round ligament and the reflection of the falciform ligament. If one dissects further along the left branch of the hepatic artery to its first bifurcation, one can often preserve the medial segment of the left lobe and carry out a resection of the lateral segment alone. Any more exact surgical resection by vascular segments is not, however, feasible.

the ligamentous attachments

The major ligamentous attachments and reflections of the liver can be identified in Figure 1-2. The *falciform ligament* is a peritoneal fold that extends from the umbilicus superiorly, contains the obliterated umbilical vein known as the round ligament and connects the liver to the anterior abdominal wall and the diaphragm.

On the posterior surface of the liver there is a bare area not covered by peritoneum but enclosed by an upper and lower layer of peritoneal reflections that contain the inferior vena cava and the hepatic veins. Surgical access to the posterior surface of the liver and these important vessels is obtained by dividing the lateral reflection and retracting the right lobe medially. The *hepatorenal ligament*, a reflection of the lower layer of the coronary ligament, passes to the upper pole of the right kidney, forming the lateral border of the

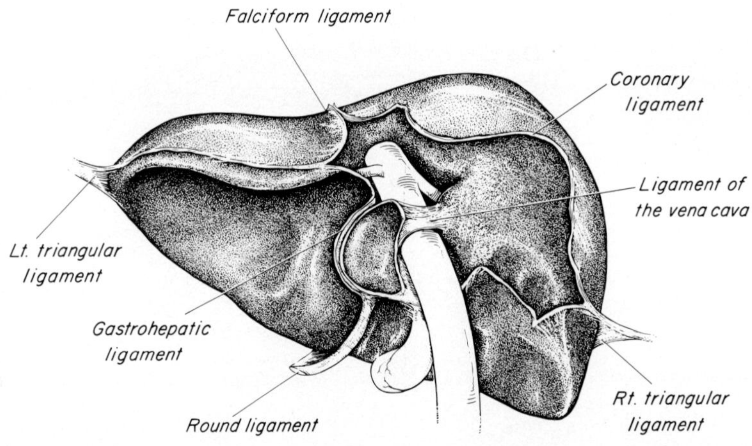

FIG. 1-2. The major ligamentous attachments of the liver

so-called hepatorenal fossa inferior and posterior to the gallbladder and gastrohepatic ligament. Division of this ligament is necessary for mobilization of the right lobe and must usually be done so that upward retraction of the right lobe will provide adequate access to the inferior vena cava during the dissection prior to the construction of a portacaval shunt. The *right triangular ligament* is the free margin of the coronary ligament. The *left triangular ligament* is continuous with the falciform ligament in front and the lesser omentum behind. These triangular ligaments form the attachments of the lobes of the liver to the under surface of the diaphragm.

lobular anatomy

A schematic cross-sectional drawing of the lobular pattern of the liver is shown in Figure 1-3. This illustrates the complex intercommunications of the vascular inflow through the hepatic artery and the portal veins with the sinusoids and thus with the central veins and the hepatic venules. The relationship of the bile ducts, their finite branches and the canaliculi can also be traced. These interdigitations are extremely complex. In addition to providing the mechanism by which the hepatic cell has access to nutrient material derived from the gut, they also identify the area where direct communication between the hepatic arterial inflow and the portal venules may occur, an arteriovenous communication that is of great importance to the

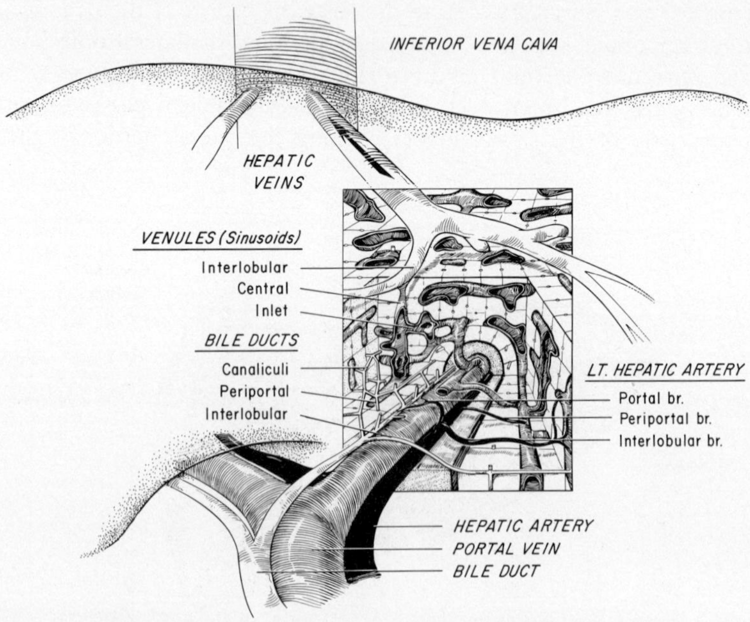

FIG. 1-3. Schematic representation of the lobular pattern of the liver

understanding of the hemodynamics of portal hypertension. Pressure and flow changes related to these communications will be discussed later under hemodynamics and the pathophysiology of portal hypertension.

vascular and biliary anatomy

Elaborate details of the blood supply of the liver and biliary tract are given in a beautiful series of descriptions and drawings by Michels; they will provide the surgeon who wishes to pursue not only the minute details of normal anatomy but the definitions of the innumerable anomalies that occur an opportunity for more information than is presented here. Only a rather cursory description of some of the more important anatomic details and more frequent anomalies will be given in this section.

portal circulation

The drawing in Figure 1-4 illustrates both the normal anatomy of the circulation with its major tributaries and the various routes of potential portal-systemic collateral channels that, in the presence of portal hypertension, provide egress of blood from the obstructed and congested splanchnic and splenic beds to the systemic venous circulation. In later sections concerned with surgical technique, reference will be made to those aspects of venous anatomy that are particu-

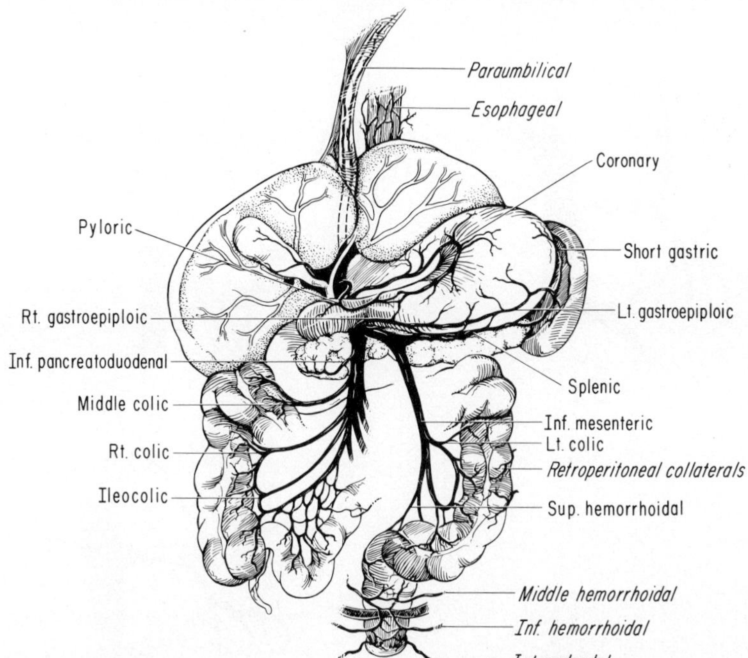

FIG. 1-4. Anatomy of the splanchnic circulation and portal-systemic collaterals

larly important and relevant to the completion of various types of surgical shunts.

hepatic arterial circulation

A precise knowledge of the hepatic arterial vascular patterns is of great importance to the surgeon operating on the liver and the upper abdominal organs, particularly the pancreas. The major variations are shown in Figures 1-5A to 1-5E; these are redrawn from Michels' descriptions based on a large series of dissections. They illustrate that what we usually consider the "normal" arterial pattern occurs in only 55 per cent of patients, and therefore one can anticipate the frequent occurrence of significant anomalies. Identification of the anatomic pattern of arterial supply to the liver is of extreme importance to

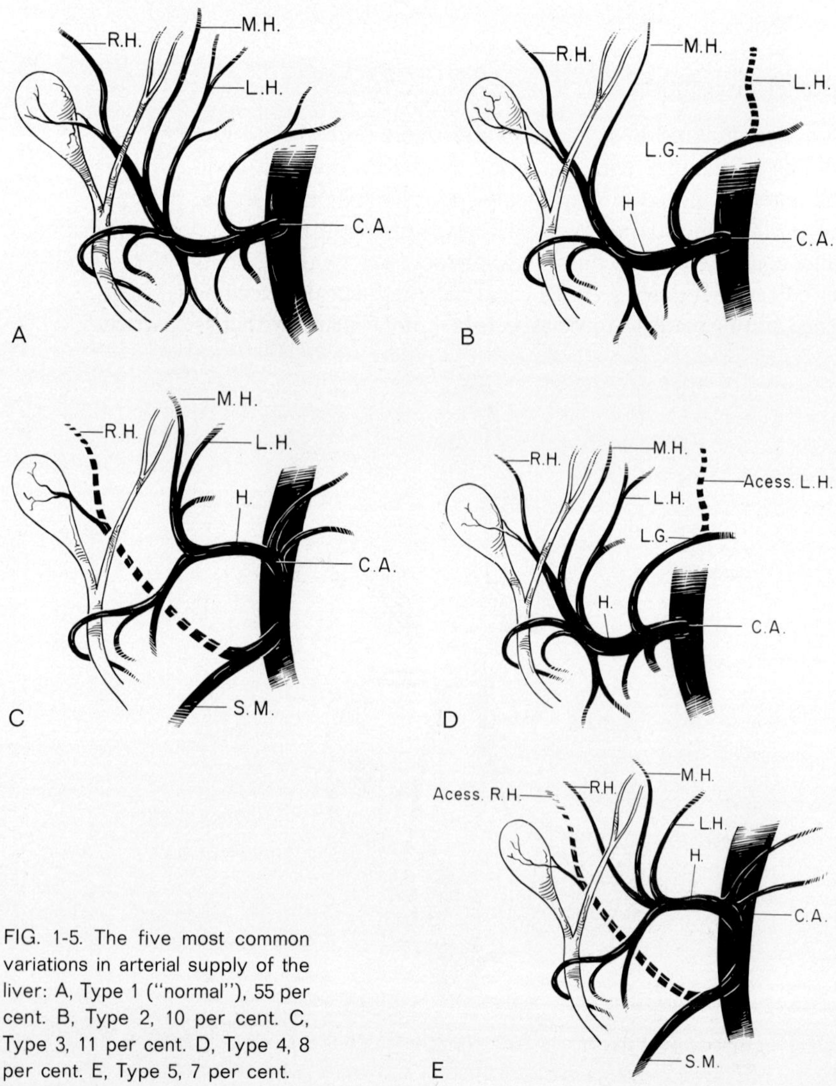

FIG. 1-5. The five most common variations in arterial supply of the liver: A, Type 1 ("normal"), 55 per cent. B, Type 2, 10 per cent. C, Type 3, 11 per cent. D, Type 4, 8 per cent. E, Type 5, 7 per cent.

the operating surgeon and is probably best defined with a selective hepatic arteriogram, a radiographic procedure that is an essential preliminary to any planned hepatic surgery. It is also vital if one is considering infusion chemotherapy, since the vascular anatomy will determine the placement of the catheter and will identify areas of the liver that may be perfused with any specific type of fluoroscopic placement. In carrying out hepatic resections it is important to identify the not infrequent occurrence of the type 3 and type 5 anomalies in which the right hepatic artery arises directly from the superior mesenteric vein. Since this anomalous origin occurs in almost one fifth of patients, it has been the cause of serious surgical problems encountered at operation. Not only in hepatic surgery but also in pancreaticoduodenectomy is it vital to recognize this particular pattern wherein the right hepatic artery passes behind the head of the pancreas and enters the liver by passing posteriorly in the gastrohepatic ligament.

hepatic veins

The venous outflow from the liver is extremely variable. There may be from three to eight small hepatic veins entering the vena cava posteriorly from the right, quadrate and caudate lobes. The main outflow from these areas of the hepatic parenchyma goes through the right hepatic vein, entering the vena cava posteriorly 2 to 4 cm. below the point where the cava passes through the diaphragm. The left hepatic veins and the blood from the left lobe usually enter the vena cava at the same level and medial to the right hepatic vein. Not infrequently, however, these two vessels become confluent within the substance of the liver and enter the vena cava posteriorly by a single trunk. It is of particular importance for the surgeon to recognize this anomaly when carrying out a right hepatic lobectomy; further reference to this anatomic feature will be made in a later chapter on the technique of hepatic resection.

the biliary system

Since this book is not directly concerned with surgery of the gallbladder, biliary tract and pancreas, no detailed reference to the normal and anomalous anatomy in these areas will be given. Certain specific references to details important to liver surgery will be made in the appropriate ensuing sections, and further reference to the superb text by Michels will provide extensive detail for any reader wishing to pursue this matter more extensively.

bibliography

Anson, B. J., and McVay, C. B.: The topographical positions and the mutual relations of the visceral branches of the abdominal aorta. A study of 100 consecutive cadavers. Anat. Rec., *67*:7–15, 1936.

Arey, L. B.: Developmental Anatomy: A Textbook and Laboratory Manual of Embryology. Ed. 6th Philadelphia, W. B. Saunders Co., 1954, 680 pp.

Browne, E. Z.: Variations in origin and course of the hepatic artery and its branches. Surgery, *8:*424–445, 1940.

Child, C. G., III: The Hepatic Circulation and Portal Hypertension. Philadelphia, W. B. Saunders Co., 1954, 444 pp.

Douglass, B. E., Baggenstoss, A. H., and Hollinshead, W. H.: The anatomy of the portal vein and its tributaries. Surg. Gynec. Obstet., *91:*562–576, 1950.

Edwards, E. A.: Functional anatomy of the porta-systemic communications. Arch. Int. Med., *88:*137–154, 1951.

Geumei, A. M., Mahfouz, M., and Aboul-Enein, A.: Intrahepatic vascular pathways. Hepatic arterioportal shunt. J. Surg. Res., *8:*463–470, 1968.

Glauser, F.: Studies on intrahepatic arterial circulation. Surgery, *33:*333–341, 1953.

Gray, H. K.: Clinical and experimental investigation of the circulation of the liver. Ann. Roy. Coll. Surg. Eng., *8:*354–365, 1951.

Hardy, K. J., and Nye, D. H.: An abnormal portal vein. Surgery *66:*676–681, 1969.

Healey, J. E., Schroy, P. C., and Sorensen, R. J.: The intrahepatic distribution of the hepatic artery in man. J. Internat. Coll. Surg., *20:*133–148, 1953.

Johns, T. N. P., and Evans, B. B.: Collateral pathways in portal hypertension. Ann. Surg., *155:*838–845, 1962.

Knisely, M. H.: Microscopic observations of the circulatory conditions in living frog liver lobules. Anat. Rec. (Suppl. 1), *73:*69–70, 1939.

Lewis, F. T.: The development of the liver. *In* Keibel, F., and Mall, F. P. (Eds.): Manual of Human Embryology. Philadelphia, J. B. Lippincott Company, 1912, vol. 2, pp. 403–445.

von Lichtenberg, F.: Portal hypertension and schistosomiasis. Ann. N.Y. Acad. Sci., *170:*100–114, 1970.

Marks, C.: Developmental basis of the portal venous system. Amer. J. Surg., *117:*671–681, 1969.

Michels, N. A.: The hepatic, cystic and retroduodenal arteries and their relations to the biliary ducts. With samples of the entire celiacal blood supply. Ann. Surg., *133:*503–524, 1951.

Michels, N. A.: Collateral arterial pathways to the liver after ligation of the hepatic artery and removal of the celiac axis. Cancer, *6:*708–724, 1953.

Reynolds, T. B.: Hepatic circulatory changes after shunt surgery. Ann. N.Y. Acad. Sci., *170:*379–391, 1970.

Rousselot, L. M., Ruzicka, F. F., and Doehner, G. A.: Portal venography via the portal and percutaneous splenic routes. Anatomic and clinical studies. Surgery, *34:*557–569, 1953.

Schwartz, S. I.: Surgical Diseases of the Liver. New York, McGraw-Hill Book Co., 1964, 387 pp.

Vennes, J. A.: Transhepatic pressure measurements. Ann. N.Y. Acad. Sci., *170:*193–201, 1970.

Wakim, K. G., and Mann, F. C.: The intrahepatic circulation of blood. Anat. Rec., *82:*233–253, 1942.

Diagnostic Techniques in Liver Surgery

CHAPTER 2

There are a number of different special techniques that have been used in assessing the microscopic picture of liver disease and of evaluating the hemodynamic changes associated with disorders of the liver and portal circulation and certain special radiologic techniques that are of particular value. Table 2-1 indicates by outline those that seem particularly appropriate to refer to in this text.

percutaneous needle biopsy

A sample of liver tissue for microscopic study can be obtained safely and with minimal discomfort by percutaneous puncture of the liver with needles designed specifically for this purpose. The Vim-Silverman needle consists of a cannula and obturator used to perforate the skin and penetrate the liver parenchyma and an inner, forked obturator that replaces the original solid obturator when the needle has been positioned properly. This forked obturator is then introduced beyond the tip of the cannula, and by twisting, a sample of liver tissue may be withdrawn that has proved very satisfactory for purposes of diagnostic microscopic evaluation of the pathology. The Menghini method employs aspiration rather than cutting. When the instrument is positioned in the hepatic parenchyma, a syringe attachment is used to draw a sample into the needle for removal and later fixation and study. The safety of either technique depends on the appropriate selection of patients, and the techniques should not be utilized in any individual with any significant defect in the clotting mechanism. The patient must be cooperative and relaxed since both techniques require him to control his respiration at the appropriate point in the procedure. Since there is a slight but definite risk of continued bleeding after needle biopsy, it should not be carried out on an ambulatory

TABLE 2-1. Diagnostic Techniques in Liver Surgery

A. Percutaneous needle biopsy
B. Hemodynamic studies
    1. Hepatic blood flow
    2. Portal pressure measurements
        a. Splenic pulp pressures
        b. Hepatic wedge pressures
        c. Transumbilical or transhepatic portal pressures
C. Radiologic techniques
    1. Esophagography
    2. Angiography (arterial and venous)
    3. Scintiscanning

basis but only in hospitalized patients who can be observed for 24 hours subsequent to the procedure. In a relatively thin patient with a large, easily palpable liver, the subcostal route may be used, but ordinarily, a transthoracic, intercostal approach in the midaxillary line in the 9th interspace is the most satisfactory. During introduction of the needle and rapid removal of the sample, the patient must control his respiration and, as mentioned above, bed rest and monitoring of vital signs for a 24 hour period are essential.

hemodynamic studies

In a subsequent chapter on the hemodynamics of portal hypertension, reference will be made in more detail to measurements of hepatic blood flow and their significance. Briefly, the principles of measurement depend on the clearance by the reticuloendothelial system of the liver of an isotopically labeled colloid (usually either gold or chromic phosphate) or by continuous drip of Bromsulphalein (BSP), which is cleared by the hepatocytes and wherein determination of flow depends on utilization of the Fick principle with measurements peripherally and in the outflow tracts.

Portal pressure measurements will also be referred to in considerably more detail and their significance in the assessment of the hemodynamics of portal hypertension evaluated in a subsequent chapter. Percutaneous introduction of a needle into the spleen through the 9th interspace in the midaxillary line on the left will permit a direct measurement of pressure that correlates very well with recorded pressures in the portal vein at the time of operation. This can be done at the same time as splenoportography; it has been used by Rousselot in particular as a diagnostic technique in the emergency ward in patients with upper gastrointestinal bleeding. Relatively few patients bleed from esophageal varices until the portal pressure exceeds 30 cm. of water. This particular test has immediate diagnostic value in the differential diagnosis of patients with upper gastrointestinal hemorrhage.

hepatic wedge pressure

The introduction of a flexible cardiac catheter through a vein in the upper extremity into the right atrium, thence into the inferior vena cava and finally into a hepatic vein permits direct sampling for both hemodynamic and biochemical measurements. If the catheter is introduced as far as possible into the hepatic venous outflow, a wedge pressure can then be obtained which is thought to represent sinusoidal pressure and corresponds to some degree with pressures in the portal vein. This latter correlation, however, requires further assessment since in patients with presinusoidal block, which is so characteristic of the portal hypertension of schistosomiasis, the portal pressure is much higher than the wedge hepatic and sinusoidal pressures. This differential may be of value in estimating in a rough way the degree of prograde flow in the portal vein and thus as an index of the metabolic effects of a surgical shunt. Confirmation of this speculation would require, however, a large series of measurements in patients with varying types of portal hypertension and a correlation with operative pressures and postshunt metabolic changes. Direct measurements of portal pressure may be obtained by transumbilical or transhepatic introduction of a catheter into a branch of the portal system itself, and, of course, direct measurements in a peripheral vein in the splanchnic bed can be carried out at the time of operation.

radiologic techniques

These include methods of visualizing esophageal varices by upper gastrointestinal series and by various methods of portography (Fig. 2-1) as well as scintiscanning and angiography.

esophagography

An *esophagogram,* as a part of an upper gastrointestinal series, is the oldest and still one of the more useful methods of determining the presence or absence of esophageal varices (Fig. 2-2). The art of adequate demonstration by esophagography requires special techniques in terms of positioning, use of the Valsalva maneuver, composition of the barium and timing of the film in order to achieve a high degree of accuracy.

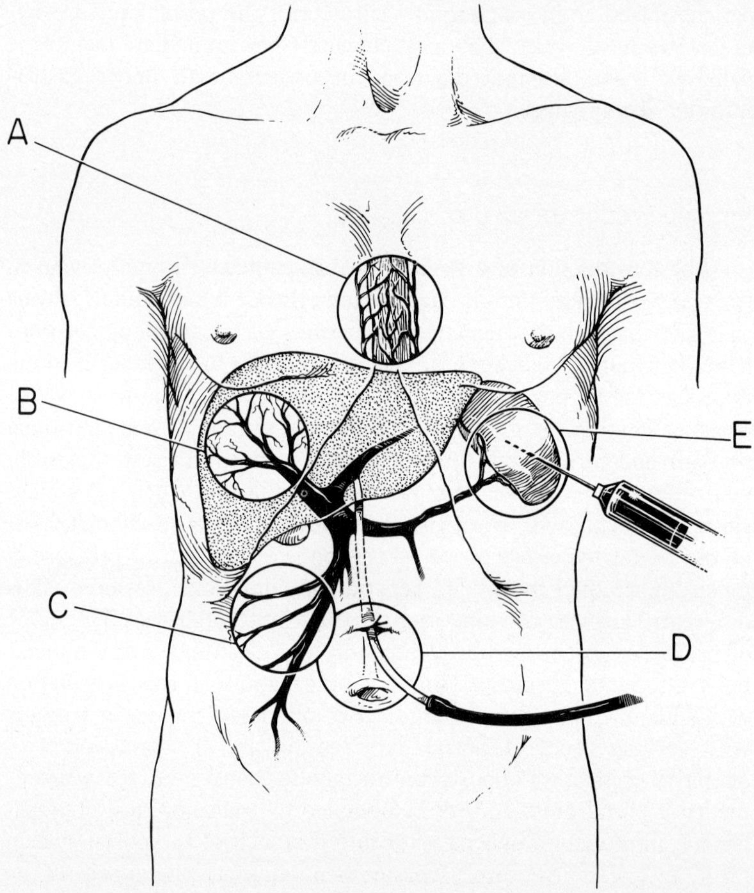

FIG. 2-1. Radiologic techniques in the diagnosis of esophageal varices. A, Esophagogram. B, Transhepatic portogram. C, Operative portogram. D, Transumbilical hepato-portogram. E, Splenoportogram.

hepatic angiography

From the early use of translumbar aortograms (Fig. 2-3) and splenoportograms, the clinical applications of abdominal angiography have been extended greatly during the past decade.

The technique of percutaneous arterial puncture, known as the Seldinger technique, has superseded the translumbar approach; with present types of sophisticated equipment, fluoroscopic techniques and improved contrast media, catheterization of visceral branches of the aorta can be carried out in all age groups (Fig. 2-4).

The procedures of selective catheterization are quite safe if one avoids these studies in patients who have severe cardiac or renal disease, specific allergies to contrast media, peripheral vascular disease or coagulation defects.

An excellent recent review of the broad area of abdominal angiography has been reported by Pollard and Nebusar. Complications of the technique were mainly technical and mechanical and included thrombus formation at the site of the introduction of the catheter, distal embolization, localized hemorrhage, the rare but reported problem of adjacent neurocompression and cerebral accidents from carotid arteriography. In Seldinger's report the mortality rate was 0.06 per cent and the incidence of serious complications 1.9 per cent.

Further discussion of angiographic techniques will be limited to those applicable to the liver. Angiographic visualization of the liver has been accomplished by the injection of dyes through a catheter placed under fluoroscopic control in the hepatic arterial, portal venous or hepatic venous routes.

Selective hepatic arteriography is probably the most valuable technique because it provides more accurate definition of the hepatic circulation, better opacification of the liver and the additional dividend of a venous phase that will usually permit at least faint visualization of the portal circulation as the dye returns from the spleen to the liver. Complication rate of hepatic arteriography is less than that of splenoportography, and this, in general, is a preferred technique if only one type of angiography is to be carried out. The accuracy of hepatic arteriography is high, with a reported 70 per cent delineation

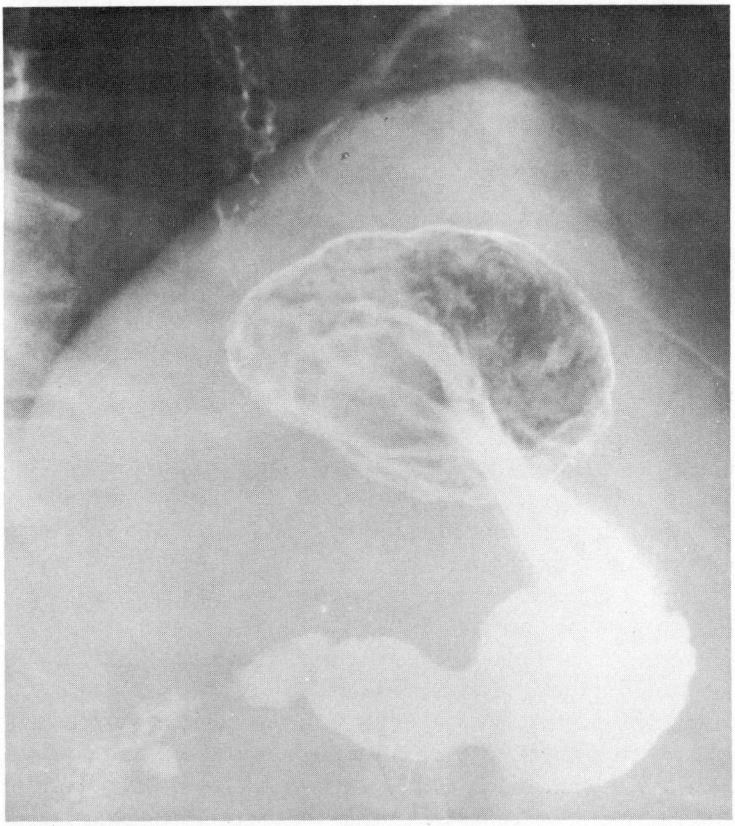

FIG. 2-2. Esophageal varices as visualized by esophagogram

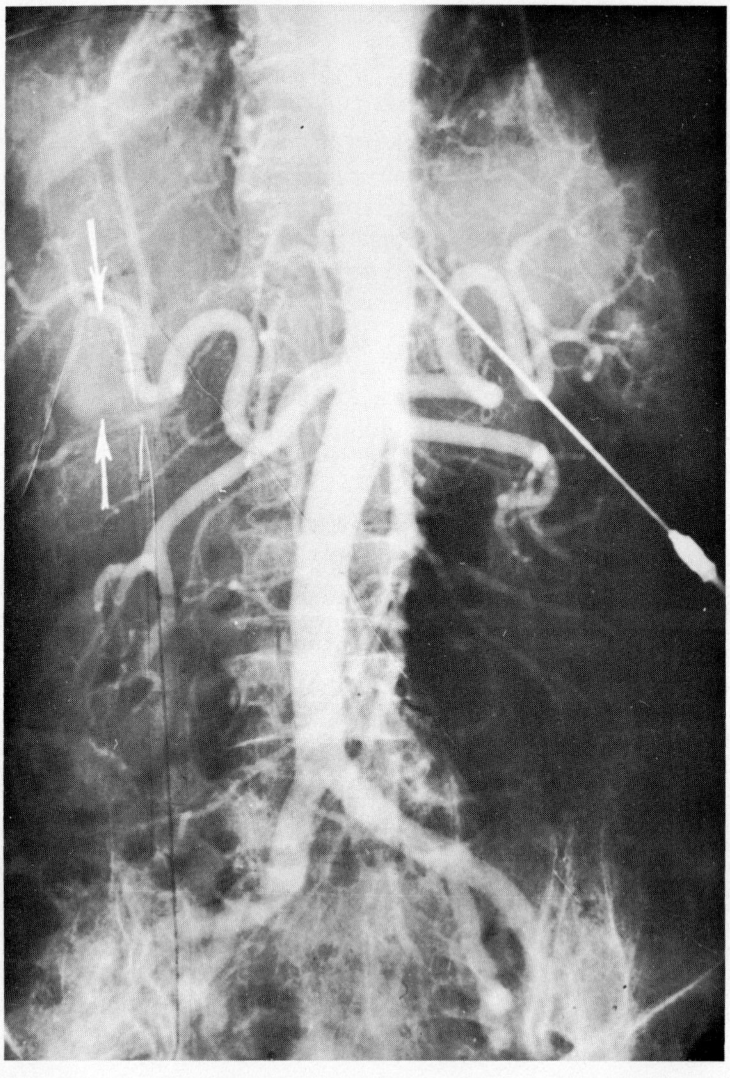

FIG. 2-3. Translumbar aortogram with localization on intrahepatic abscess

of existing tumors with relatively uncommon false positive reports. This is approximately the same degree of accuracy as has been reported for scintiscanning of the liver, and when these two techniques are combined, the overall diagnostic accuracy is further improved. *Metastatic cancer* of the liver is the most common neoplastic lesion, and when the nodules are of reasonable size or number, macroscopic tumor vessels and tumor "blush" can be visualized (Figs. 2-5A and 2-5B). When the metastases are necrotic or relatively avascular, they may appear as filling defects but are more difficult to detect than those in which tumor vessels exist. Large tumors (Figs. 2-6A and 2-6B), even if avascular, can be identified by distortion of the intrahepatic arterial pattern. When diffuse invasion of the liver by a large number of small, avascular metastases occurs, however, accurate diagnosis may

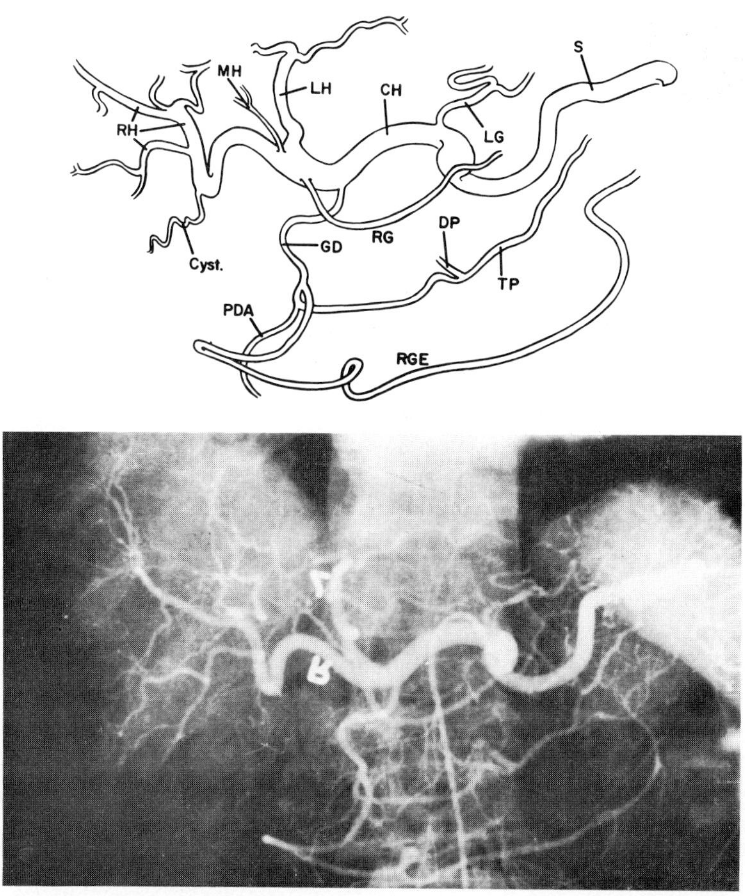

FIG. 2-4. Normal selective celiac arteriogram

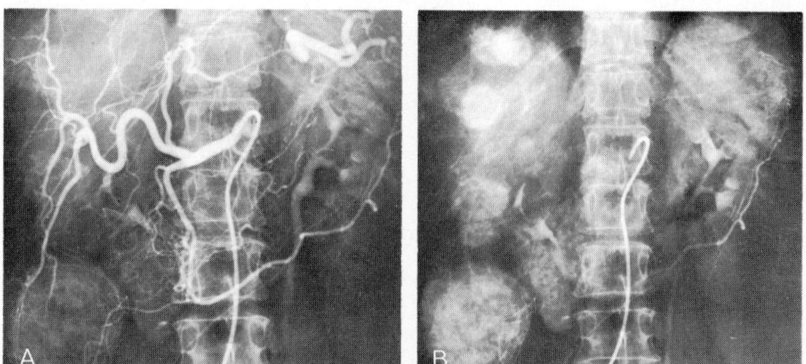

FIG. 2-5. A, Multiple metastases (carcinoid)—arterial phase. B, Multiple metastases (carcinoid)—venous phase

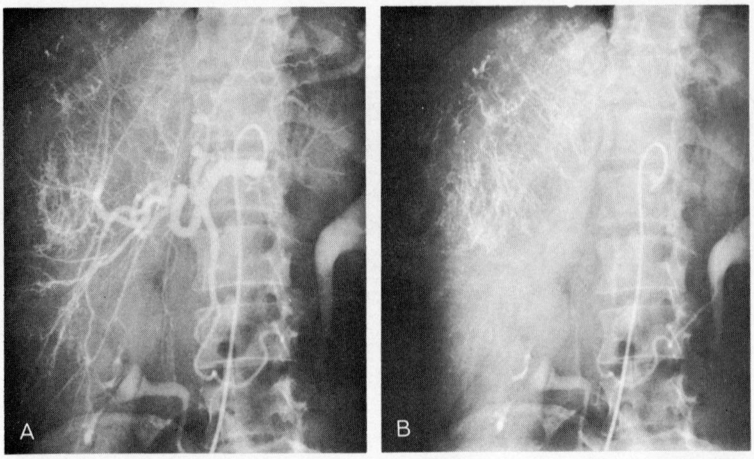

FIG. 2-6. A, Solitary metastasis (melanoma)—arterial phase. B, Solitary metastasis (melanoma)—venous phase.

be difficult, and the situation can be confused with other diffuse hepatic disease such as cirrhosis, which may also show a mottled appearance caused by diffuse areas of avascular lesions. *Primary hepatic tumors* will show arteriographic changes that vary with the specific pathologic entity. *Hepatoma,* which is the most common primary hepatic tumor, is often multinodular, but approximately a third of these tumors may be solitary and of enormous size. Only when hepatoma assumes a diffusely infiltrating form is diagnosis difficult since it may be indistinguishable from cirrhosis, as is diffuse metastatic disease of the liver. Hepatomas are ordinarily recognized by extensive abnormal vascularization, occasionally with evidence of arterial-venous shunting. Because of vascularity, these tumors will ordinarily show a dense tumor stain. *Cholangiocarcinomas* are more avascular and more difficult to detect and diagnose than hepatomas, but again, distortion of the normal vascular pattern will usually identify the presence and anatomic location of the tumor (Figs. 2-7A, 2-7B and 2-7C). *Hemangiomatous tumors* are almost always benign and are readily detectable because of their extreme vascularity. Radiographic diagnostic subtleties may make it possible to distinguish hemangioma from a very vascular hepatoma, but this distinction may require a high degree of sophistication. *Cysts* and other benign tumors are delineated by distortion of the normal vasculature.

DIFFUSE, NON-NEOPLASTIC DISEASE OF THE LIVER. Changes in the vasculature of the liver reflect the severity, extent, stage and form of cirrhosis. In *advanced cirrhosis,* the hepatic arteries may enlarge as the proportion of the liver blood flow supplied by the arterial inflow begins to exceed that of the portal vein. Within the liver itself, a characteristic corkscrew pattern (Fig. 2-8) may develop, but since this is caused by chronic destruction of hepatic parenchyma, it may be seen with any diffuse fibrotic process within the liver.

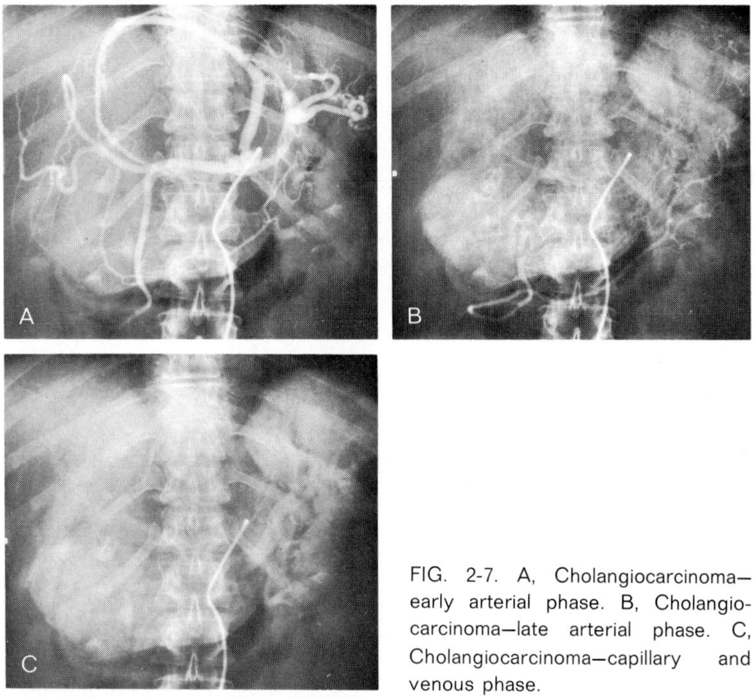

FIG. 2-7. A, Cholangiocarcinoma—early arterial phase. B, Cholangiocarcinoma—late arterial phase. C, Cholangiocarcinoma—capillary and venous phase.

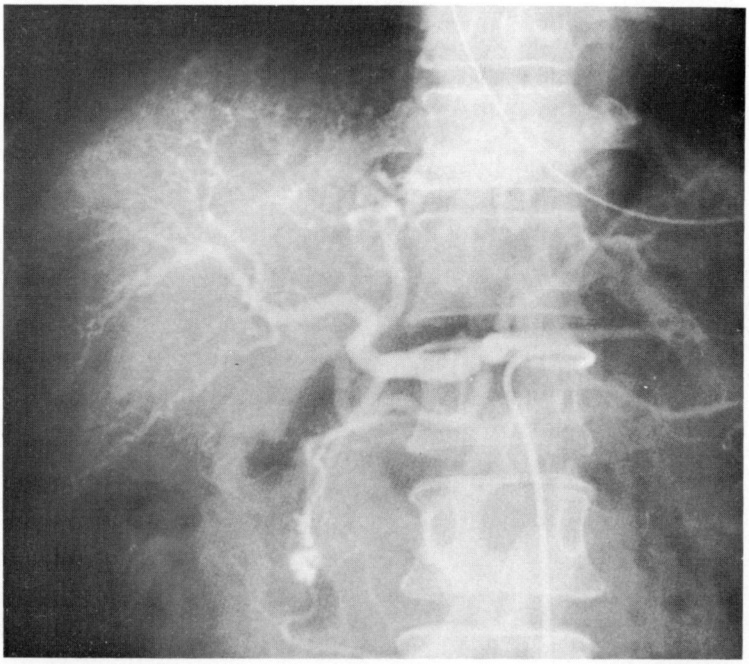

FIG. 2-8. Cirrhosis of the liver showing typical pattern of corkscrew arteries

During the venous phase, the hepatic veins may show tortuosity, narrowing and irregularities. *Hepatic trauma* may be diagnosed in terms of existence, location and extent by hepatic arteriography. Localized accumulation of the contrast medium in areas of the liver, extravasation into a bile duct, a space-occupying defect such as a subcapsular hematoma and sometimes extravasation of the dye into the peritoneal cavity may often confirm the existence of suspected traumatic injury. The catastrophic nature of serious hepatic injury often limits utilization of this radiographic technique, but if the patient's condition is stable and liver injury is suspected, this technique combined with splenic arteriography can be extremely helpful in cases of diffuse abdominal injury.

PORTAL VENOGRAPHY. Opacification of the portal venous system may be carried out through percutaneous introduction of dye into the spleen, into the liver itself, by identification, dilatation and introduction of a catheter through the umbilical vein into the left portal vein or by direct injection at operation into one of the splanchnic branches of the portal circulation (see Fig. 2-1). Any of these techniques can be used appropriately to delineate the anatomy, identify the existence and frequently the extent of an extrahepatic portal bed block, demonstrate the presence of esophageal varices and indicate the patency of surgically constructed portal-systemic shunts. The most frequently used technique has been *splenoportography* (Fig. 2-9), the main complication of which is postinjection bleeding. For this reason, it has been our practice to carry out splenoportography only when the patient is ready for whatever operative procedure may be indicated. Thus, if a shunt is indicated and postpuncture bleeding occurs, splenectomy and construction of a splenorenal shunt can be carried out immediately. One major source of diagnostic error in this technique is the confusion sometimes projected by the laminar flow in the portal vein, which may suggest a partially occluding thrombus. Stagnation or reversal of flow in the portal vein may give the false impression of an extrahepatic portal bed block. In fact, this technique has been used by Warren and others to estimate the extent of hepatofugal flow in an attempt to predict the likelihood of postshunt encephalopathy; this particular problem will be discussed in more detail in a subsequent chapter. *Transhepatic venography* is a technique whereby access to a branch of the portal vein may be achieved by percutaneous introduction of a needle into the liver; this approach has limited usefulness and has not had widespread application.

TRANSUMBILICAL VENOGRAPHY (Fig. 2-10). Access to the left branch of the portal vein is possible by surgical identification of the obliterated umbilical vein just above the navel with subsequent dilatation and catheterization. This technique has been used not only for angiography but also for the procurement of physiologic and biochemical information and for temporary or permanent (rarely) decompression of portal hypertension.

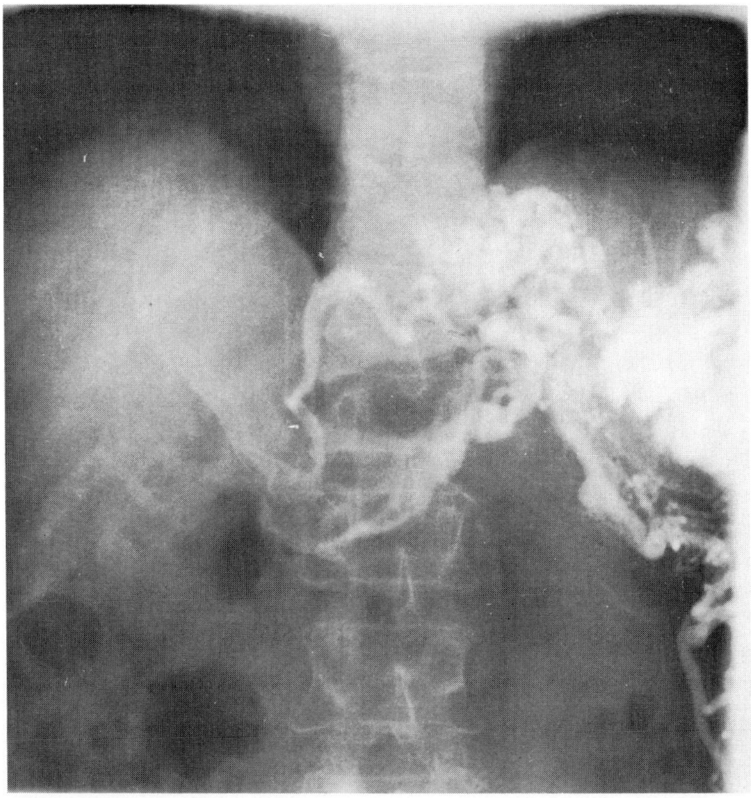

FIG. 2-9. Splenoportogram demonstrating extrahepatic portal bed block with collateral channels to the liver and extensive gastric and esophageal varices

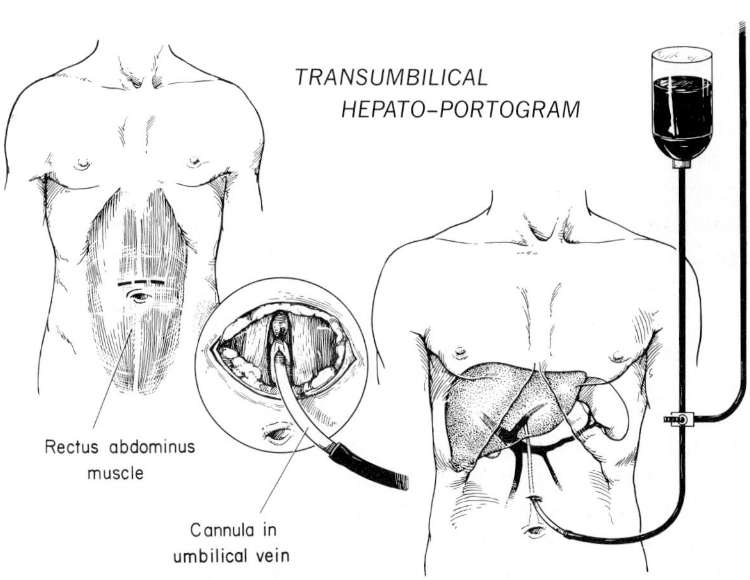

FIG. 2-10. Technique of transumbilical portography

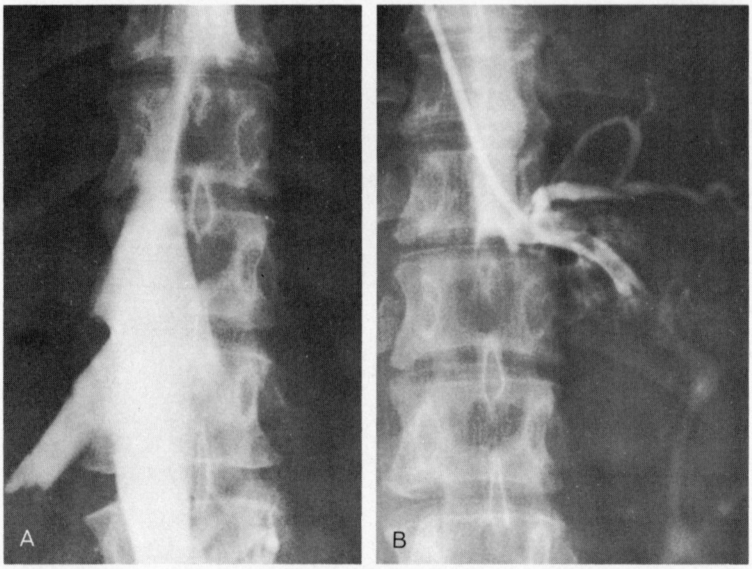

FIG. 2-11. A, Cavogram with compression of interior vena cava from polycystic liver. B, Hepatic venogram phase—polycystic liver with thrombus in left hepatic vein.

HEPATIC VENOGRAPHY (Figs. 2-11A and 2-11B). Catheterization of the hepatic veins with manometric studies and associated venography is sometimes a valuable technique, particularly if a Budd-Chiari syndrome is suspected. Unfortunately, failure to catheterize or visualize the hepatic veins may be caused by technical difficulties rather than the existence of occlusion, but certainly if the hepatic veins can be successfully visualized, this particular source of postsinusoidal block can be eliminated. Suprahepatic sources of hepatic congestion such as narrowing of the vena cava as it passes through the diaphragm, congenital anomalies or obstruction from retroperitoneal malignant disease can be demonstrated in the retrohepatic vena cava. The technique of hepatic vein catheterization may assume greater importance in the future because of increasing evidence that thorough evaluation of abnormal hemodynamics of portal hypertension may be essential in selecting patients for shunt surgery. The ability to obtain both physiologic information and anatomic visualization is important not only in suspected outflow obstruction but also in defining those patients in whom a normal wedge hepatic pressure in the presence of portal hypertenison may indicate either an extrahepatic portal bed block or a specific presinusoidal block such as occurs in idiopathic periportal fibrosis, in schistosomiasis and in certain types of cirrhosis in which extensive destruction of hepatic parenchyma has not occurred. Again, further discussion of the hemodynamics of portal hypertension will be presented in a subsequent chapter.

scintiscan of the liver

By injection of radioisotopes that localize in the liver, an outline of it may be reproduced that will give an indication of its size and configuration, demonstrate the size and location of intrahepatic tumors, abscesses or cysts, show a fairly characteristic pattern on extrahepatic biliary obstruction and, by certain specific techniques, distinguish between obstructive and intrahepatic causes of jaundice (Fig. 2-12).

DEFINITION OF TECHNIQUES. *Radioactive Colloid.* The use of radioactive colloidal gold (^{198}Au) or technetium sulfur colloid (^{99M}Tc sulfur colloid) is based on phagocytosis of the particles by the reticuloendothelial (R-E; Kupffer) cells in the liver that line the hepatic sinusoids. Since the liver is a major locus of the R-E cells of the body and since about 40 per cent of the cardiac output per minute goes through the liver, an excellent image may be reproduced during the half-life of the radionuclide.

^{131}*I-Rose Bengal.* This particular dye follows the same pathways as Bromsulphalein and is cleared by the hepatic parenchymal cells from blood traversing the liver. It is then, as is Bromsulphalein, excreted through the bile canaliculi into the extrahepatic biliary system and eventually reaches the intestinal tract in the absence of obstruction. It is therefore an extremely useful agent not only for outlining the liver itself and defining areas of intrahepatic disease but also in distinguishing between intrahepatic causes of jaundice and extrahepatic biliary obstruction.

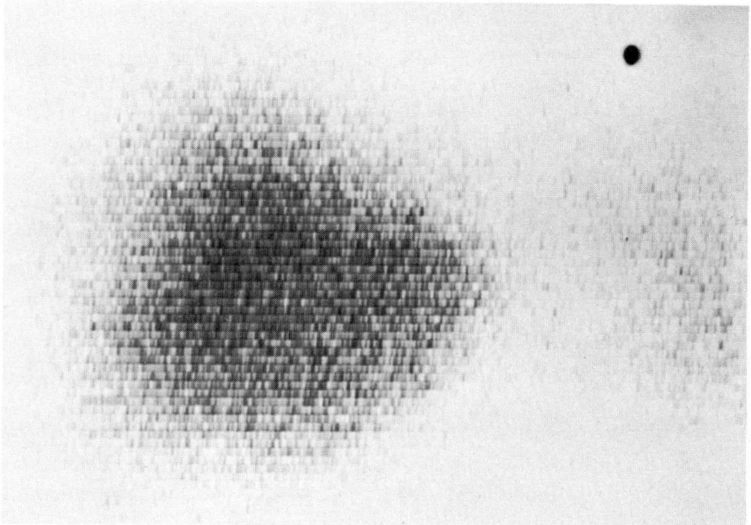

FIG. 2-12. Scintiscan of normal liver

Iodinated Human Serum Albumin (*^{131}I-Albumin*). Clearance of this particular agent is dependent also on hepatic function but is an indication of the vascular supply of the liver or of lesions within the liver and therefore may be particularly useful in the definition of unusually vascular tumors. It serves also to outline the major hepatic sinusoidal distribution.

METHODS. *Static Anatomic Imaging.* This can probably be best obtained by the intravenous administration of a short-lived agent such as ^{99M}Tc sulfur colloid in dosages of 1 to 3 mc. This particular technique is probably most frequently used today. An equally satisfactory scan may be obtained with ^{198}Au, but because of the longer physical half-life and the beta emission, a much smaller dose is recommended and, in that sense, technetium sulfur colloid is preferable.

Hepatic Excretion Studies. ^{131}I-rose bengal is administered with an intravenous dose of 3 mμCi. per kg. Not only will this give a satisfactory outline of the liver and define intrahepatic lesions, but by counts obtained elsewhere in the body, hepatic excretion rate of the dye may be estimated. Since the particular usefulness of this isotope is in determining the patency of the biliary tract, the abdominal area below the liver should be included in the study. In utilizing rose bengal in the differential diagnosis of jaundice, one must correlate the disappearance rate from the blood with the presence or absence of radioactivity in the abdominal area below the liver. With a patent biliary tract, one might anticipate the prompt appearance of radioactivity in the intestinal tract although some forms of severe intrahepatic cholestasis may impede the excretion of rose bengal and make the differential less clear cut. Delayed studies, including a 24 hour scan, should be obtained before any final diagnosis of total biliary obstruction is made.

Hepatic Blood Pool Studies. The use of ^{131}I human serum albumin is most helpful as a supplementary test following a scan with one of the radioactive colloids. After intravenous administration in a dose of 3 mμCi. per kg., sufficient activity appears in liver sinusoids so that an image can be obtained within a few minutes of injection. Blood pool scans of the liver with this agent can help in clarifying the nature of some of the focal defects seen in the colloid scans. Sometimes intense activity may be demonstrated in a lesion that was "cold" on the colloid scan.

GENERAL CONSIDERATIONS. Scintiscans, by use of the various techniques described, are extremely useful in definition of the size and configuration of the liver, in delineation of focal intrahepatic disease, in definition of diffuse hepatic disease, in identification of extrahepatic lesions such as subphrenic abscess when the liver scan is combined with one of the lungs or when the scan is superimposed anatomically on a standard radiographic film, and as an aid in distinguishing between intrahepatic and extrahepatic causes of jaundice.

These relatively simple techniques are of value in recording the regeneration of the liver after major hepatic resection and following the changes in intrahepatic disease over a period of days or weeks when it is not considered advisable to carry out a surgical exploration. Sequential studies may well clarify the nature of the lesion and avoid unnecessary surgery. Examples of the types of conditions demonstrable by scintiscanning are shown in Figure 2-13A to 2-13F.

The scintiscan is, however, not infallible in diagnosis of disease of the liver, and particularly in the delineation of focal lesions, it is best used in combination with selective arteriography.

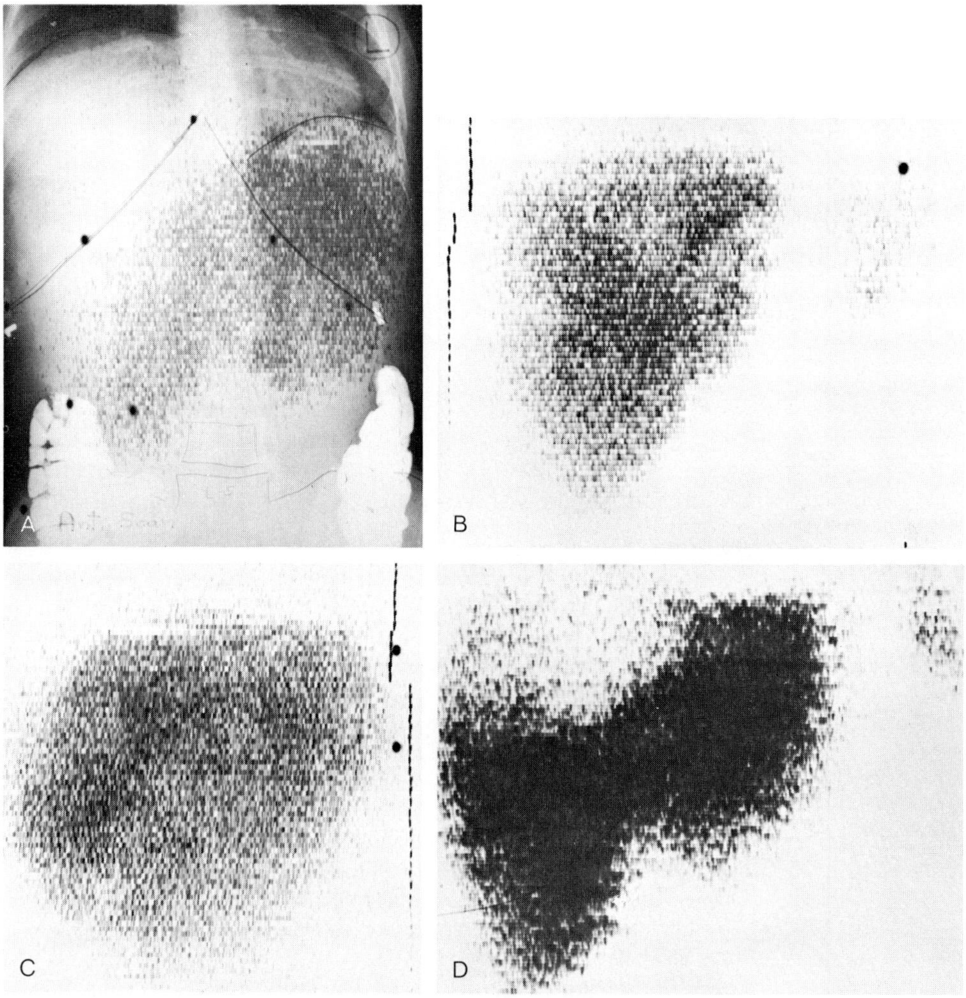

FIG. 2-13. A, Scintiscan. Solitary cystic hepatoma, right lobe of liver. B, Scintiscan. Multiple nodules of metastatic cancer (anterior view). C, Scintiscan. Multiple nodules of metastatic cancer (lateral view). D, Scintiscan. Liver abscess, right lobe of liver.

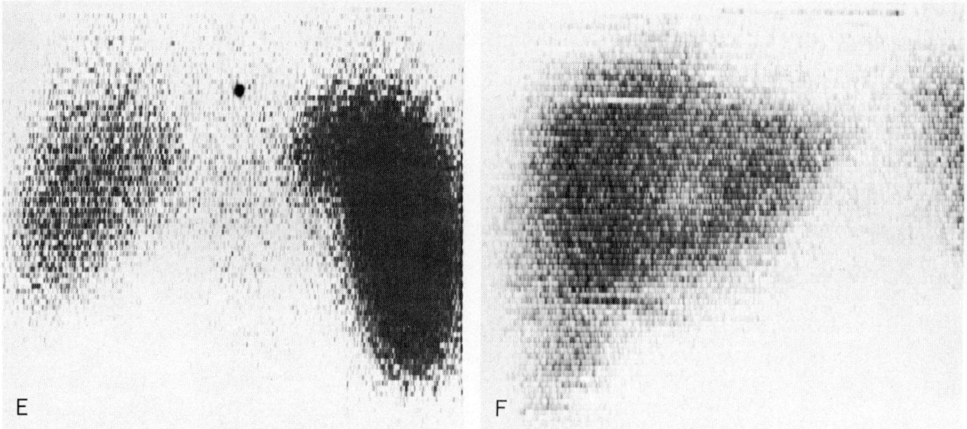

FIG. 2-13. E, Scintiscan. Cirrhosis of the liver, portal hypertension and splenomegaly. F, Scintiscan. Biliary obstruction from carcinoma of the pancreas and dilatation of common bile duct (showing as a filling defect)

bibliography

general

Hermann, R. E., and Hoerr, S. O.: Aids in the diagnosis of traumatic hemobilia. Surg. Gynec. Obstet., *125:*55–58, 1967.

Warren, W. D., and Muller, W. H., Jr.: A clarification of some hemodynamic changes in cirrhosis and their surgical significance. Ann. Surg., *150:* 413–427, 1959.

angiography and venography

Baum, S., Roy, R., Finkelstein, A. K., and Blakemore, W. S.: Clinical application of selective celiac and superior mesenteric arteriography. Radiology, *84:*279–295, 1965.

Boijsen, E.: Selective angiography of the celiac axis and superior mesenteric artery in cirrhosis of the liver. Rev. Int. Hepat., *15:*323–336, 1965.

Boijsen, E., and Ekman, C.-A.: Angiography in portal hypertension. J. Cardiov. Surg., (Suppl. *6*):45–50, 1965.

Boijsen, E., Ekman, C.-A., and Olin, T.: Coeliac and superior mesenteric angiography in portal hypertension. Acta Chir. Scand., *126:*315–325, 1963.

Boijsen, E., Judkins, M. P., and Simay, A.: Angiographic diagnosis of hepatic rupture. Radiology, *86:*66–72, 1966.

Lavoie, P., et al.: The umbilicoportal approach for the study of splanchnic circulation: Technical, radiological and hemodynamic considerations. Canad. J. Surg., *9:*338–343, 1966.

Leevy, C. M., and Gliedman, M. L.: Practical and research value of hepatic-vein catheterization. New Eng. J. Med., *258:*696–700; 738–743, 1958.

Machado, A. L., Martins, J. M., Lima, G. B., y Dourado, I. F.: Cateterismo das veias hepáticas. Rev. Ass. Med. Brasil, *9:*73–79, 1963.

Nebesar, R. A., and Pollard, J. J.: Portal venography by selective arterial catheterization. Amer. J. Roentgen., *97:*477–487, 1966.

Nebesar, R. A., Pollard, J. J., Edmunds, L. H., Jr., and McKhann, C. F.: Indications for selective celiac and superior mesenteric angiography. Experience with 128 cases. Amer. J. Roentgen., *92:*1100–1109, 1964.

Panke, W. F., et al.: Technique, hazards, and usefulness of percutaneous splenic portography. J. A. M. A. *169:*1032–1037, 1959.

Pollard, J. J., and Nebesar, R. A.: Altered hemodynamics in the Budd-Chiari syndrome demonstrated by selective hepatic and selective splenic angiography. Radiology, *89:*236–243, 1967.

Pollard, J. J., and Nebesar, R. A.: Abdominal angiography. New Eng. J. Med., *279:*1035–1042; 1093–1100; 1148–1152, 1968.

Pollard, J. J., Nebesar, R. A., and Mattoso, L. F.: Angiographic diagnosis of benign diseases of the liver. Radiology, *86:*276–283, 1966.

Steichen, F. M., and Sheiner, N. M.: Traumatic intrahepatic hemobilia. Arch. Surg., *92:*838–847, 1966.

Stone, H. H., Jordan, W. D., Acker, J. J., and Martin, J. D., Jr.: Portal arteriovenous fistulas. Review and case report. Amer. J. Surg., *109:* 191–196, 1965.

Stulberg, H. J., and Bierman, H. R.: Selective hepatic arteriography. Normal anatomy, anatomic variations, and pathological conditions. Radiology, *85:*46–55, 1965.

radioisotope scanning

Gollin, F. F., Sims, J. L., and Cameron, J. R.: Liver scanning and liver function tests. A comparative study. J. A. M. A., *187:*111–116, 1964.

Lum, C. H., Marshall, W. J., Kozoll, D. D., and Meyer, K. A.: The use of radioactive (I^{131}-labeled) rose bengal in the study of human liver disease: Its correlation with liver function tests. Ann. Surg., *149:*353–367, 1959.

Nagler, W., Bender, M. A., and Blau, M.: Radioisotope photo-scanning of the liver. Gastroenterology, *44:*36–43, 1963.

Wilson, F. E., Preston, D. F., and Overholt, E. L.: Detection of hepatic neoplasm. Hepatic scanning combined with liver-function studies. J. A. M. A., *209:*676–679, 1969.

Hemodynamics and Pathophysiology of Portal Hypertension

CHAPTER 3

history

From the early recorded observations relating to human biology, it is clear that the liver assumed particular importance in a number of civilizations. Galen attributed a number of functions to this large and obviously important organ including the formation of blood, the origin of animal heat, the source of the veins of the body and of a number of mythical humors relating to human disease and behavior. Many of these misconceptions have persisted in our language in terms such as "melancholy" and "choleric" (Fig. 3-1). Both Fabricius and Vesalius described the portal vein with anatomic precision and contributed to exposing the omniscient and fanciful errors that Galen had perpetuated. Until Harvey described the circulation of the blood in 1628, however, there was no important insight into the nature or even the direction of portal flow. Some 25 years after Harvey's impressive studies on the circulation, Glisson initiated the present understanding of the physiology and hemodynamics of the liver when he perfused the portal vein with thin milk introduced through a goose quill and observed not only the flow through the liver to the vena cava and eventually to the heart and lungs but also noted the fine reticular distribution beneath the capsule that bears his name, thus demonstrating both the venous and lymphatic channels in the liver.

According to the work of Oré, Schiff and others in animals, ligation of the portal vein appeared to be invariably fatal, and death was attributed to deprivation of portal blood. Claude Bernard, correct in this instance as in so many others, suspected that death was caused by pooling of the splanchnic blood, but it was Eck in his classic

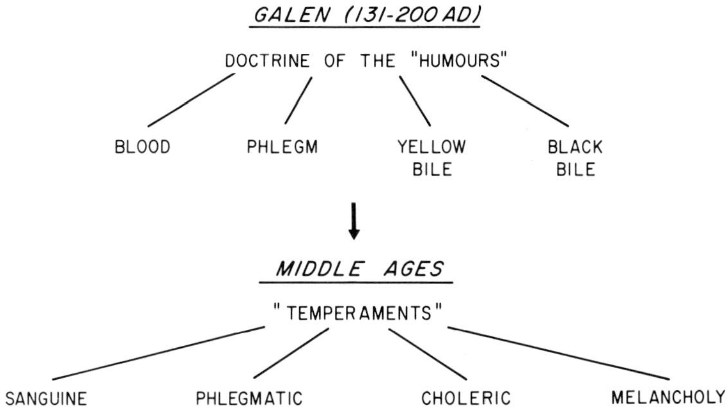

FIG. 3-1. Concept of "humours" as derived from Galen and subsequent medieval writings

although distinctly limited experiments who demonstrated that survival of the animal was possible after complete diversion of portal blood. The portacaval shunt that bears his name, consisting of a side-to-side anastomosis and ligation of the portal vein on the hepatic side, was carried out on eight dogs, of whom one died immediately after operation and six others between two and seven days postoperatively. One animal lived in apparently good health for two and one-half months before escaping from the somewhat limited surveillance in the laboratory, never to be seen again. Since Eck himself left for military service and made no further contributions to the medical literature, the eponym that is so familiar to those interested in the portal circulation rests entirely on a single, short article by one man reporting one reasonably long term survivor among eight experimental animals. Although Eck made no specific observations beyond noting the survival of this one dog, subsequent observers and investigators have filled the medical literature with experimental and clinical observations on the biochemical and hemodynamic effects of this type of portal diversion, both in the normal physiologic state and in various types of experimental conditions and human disease. More on this subject will be included in later chapters.

The feasibility of constructing a portacaval shunt in man for the relief of portal hypertension was demonstrated by the pioneering work of Whipple. Later we were able to show that resections of the portal vein for invasive carcinoma of the pancreas with the construction of a superior mesenteric-caval shunt were compatible with survival although attended by complex metabolic disorders.

Child clarified very nicely the early misconceptions relating to ligation of the portal vein by pointing out the significant species difference that exists. Although the dog and other laboratory animals will die within a few hours after ligation of the portal vein because of pooling of blood in the splanchnic bed, the same procedure in monkeys and in man does not produce the same lethal result, presumably because of the more extensive natural portal-systemic shunts in the primate.

the normal portal circulation

hepatic blood flow

During the past few years two methods have been utilized to measure the total blood flow to the liver. BSP clearance technique, which employs the Fick principle, is somewhat unsatisfactory because of the requirements of catheterization of the hepatic vein and also because many circumstances in health and disease will alter the venous concentration of the dye and introduce the possibility of an erroneous extraction ratio. Both radioactive colloidal gold and chromic phosphate labeled with ^{32}P have been employed by a number of investigators with varying and sometimes contradictory results. The amount of radioactivity administered is small in both instances, thus permitting frequent measurements without risk; neither technique requires catheterization. These methods utilize the principle of the disappearance of radioactivity from the blood since both these substances are cleared totally by passage through the liver. These techniques are not completely satisfactory either, particularly in the presence of the complex vascular changes that occur with intrahepatic portal bed block. Both the colloidal gold and chromic phosphate are removed by the spleen as well as the liver, thus introducing the possibility of error unless the total splenic flow perfuses the liver as it does under normal circumstances. With the development of collateral circulation from both the splenic and splanchnic circulations, an undetermined amount of the blood initially entering the bed from which the portal flow normally derives will escape prior to actual passage through the liver or even through the spleen and return to the systemic circulation. In spite of the potential errors and discrepancies in reported values, these techniques have been useful in clarifying some of the hemodynamic problems of the portal circulation.

There has been too little experience as yet with the technique of the washout of isotopic xenon to comment on its usefulness or accuracy in the study of the total hepatic blood flow.

In general, normal values of estimated hepatic blood flow derived from disappearance curves in the peripheral blood indicate that about 1800 cc. or 40 per cent of the total cardiac output perfuses the liver per minute. While there is considerable agreement among various investigators on the amount of normal liver blood flow, tremendous variation and considerable discrepancy have been noted in efforts to follow the changes occurring under diverse circumstances of intrahepatic disease. Further discussion of these complicated changes will be found later.

Of the total liver blood flow in the normal individual, about 75 per cent is contributed by the portal vein, which carries blood of about

80 per cent oxygen saturation, thus contributing between 40 and 50 per cent of the total oxygen supply from the liver if extraction ratios can be interpreted properly.

normal portal pressure

Pressures in both health and disease have been recorded utilizing direct measurements at operation, intrahepatic measurements by means of a percutaneous catheter, splenic pulp pressures and hepatic wedge pressures (which have been well accepted as representing sinusoidal levels). Of great interest and significance have been the measurements in portal hypertension at varying points in the open and occluded portal vein. The terminology introduced by Warren is very satisfactory and is best defined by the diagram in Figure 3-2 indicating our modifications of his concept. A free portal pressure (FPP) is self-evident. The hepatic occluded portal pressure (HOPP) refers to measurements taken on the hepatic side of an occluded portal vein, and the peripheral occluded pressure (POPP) refers to the pressure in the splanchnic bed when the portal vein is occluded. Although these values will change with variations from the resting state, the following figures are, in general, accepted as the average normal range and are recorded in centimeters of saline: FPP = 15 to 20; HOPP = 5 to 10; POPP = 40 to 60. This information should serve as a base line for discussing the complex changes that occur with varying types of portal hypertension.

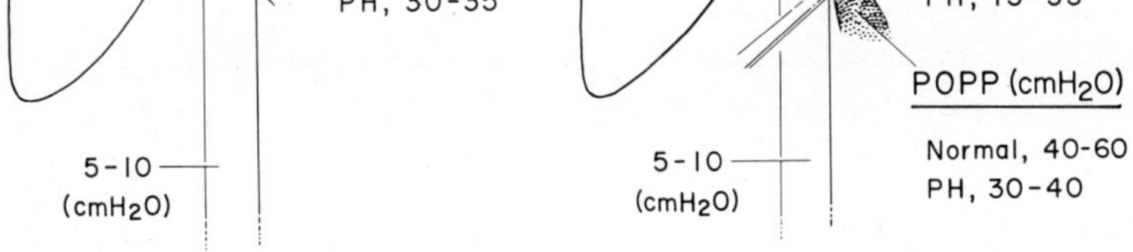

FIG. 3-2. Diagram of hepatic pressure recordings (modified from Warren and Zeppa)

pharmacology and the portal circulation

Although many pharmacologic agents such as epinephrine and norepinephrine have effects on the hemodynamics of the portal circulation, the only one that is of clinical significance at the moment is vasopressin (surgical Pituitrin). Studies under normal conditions in animals and confirmed by various observations in man indicate that this drug has a depressor effect on portal venous pressure with a fall of about 40 per cent lasting some 20 to 30 minutes after infusion. This would appear to be brought about by a direct constrictor action on the arterioles and capillaries and associated with a decrease in the splanchnic and hepatic blood flow. This decrease in the intrahepatic flow, however, appears to be compensated for by increased hepatic oxygen extraction so that oxygen consumption remains the same. The overall pharmacologic action of vasopressin results in a redistribution of blood flow with a diversion primarily from the splanchnic bed but also from the kidneys and skin, and it is associated with some degree of coronary vasoconstriction. This long recognized depressor effect on the portal circulation has been utilized therapeutically in the management of portal hypertension with bleeding esophageal varices; it will be referred to in more detail in subsequent chapters relative to clinical problems.

pathophysiology in portal hypertension and the effect of shunts

Since a wide variety of abnormalities develops secondary to different types of portal bed block in the portal circulation itself, within the liver or in the outflow channels leading from the sinusoids, extraordinarily complex and varied patterns of hemodynamic changes may occur. It has become increasingly apparent that logical classification and interpretation of these changes are essential if the proper therapeutic procedure is to be selected for the correction of the complications of portal hypertension. The accumulation of experimental and clinical information relative to changes in flow and pressure under varying circumstances has increased our understanding to some degree but has not, as yet, led to any infallible analysis of available information or completely accurate assessment of the type of procedure to be selected for each individual case. In this section a review will be made of the changes both in hepatic blood flow and in portal hemodynamics that have led to a better classification of portal hypertension and hopefully to more reasonable surgical approaches.

CHANGES IN LIVER BLOOD FLOW. With utilization of the techniques described above, a rather controversial amount of information has been collected on liver blood flow under conditions of portal hypertension. This might be expected because of the diversity of the changes caused in the liver by various cirrhotic processes. There is a wide variation in recorded data on liver blood flow in cirrhosis. Many cases fall well within the normal range while others will show very significant decreases of up to 50 per cent in estimated hepatic blood flow. Somewhat surprisingly, the initial measurement of hepatic blood flow has not been very effective as a predictor of the course of any given patient relative to shunt surgery; it would appear that changes in hepatic blood flow brought about by a shunt are more significant than the actual preoperative level.

In experimental animals complete diversion of portal blood from the liver through a portacaval shunt results in a 40 per cent decrease in liver blood flow (Fig. 3-3). In this type of experimental preparation, as in man under similar conditions (resection of the portal vein for carcinoma of the pancreas), the operation is invariably followed by serious encephalopathy and usually by progressive deterioration in hepatic function with a very high mortality over the months after operation. If, however, liver blood flow is maintained, either permanently by portacaval or renoportal (Fig. 3-4) transposition or temporarily by periarterial neurectomy, the immediate effects of the Eck fistula do not occur (Fig. 3-5). Thus, it would appear that many of the complications of portal-systemic shunting are related as much to the serious alterations in liver blood flow as to the actual diversion of portal blood around the liver.

These observations are, however, only indirectly applicable to patients with cirrhosis of the liver since it has been shown by Nardi, Warren and others that even a complete diversion by end-to-side

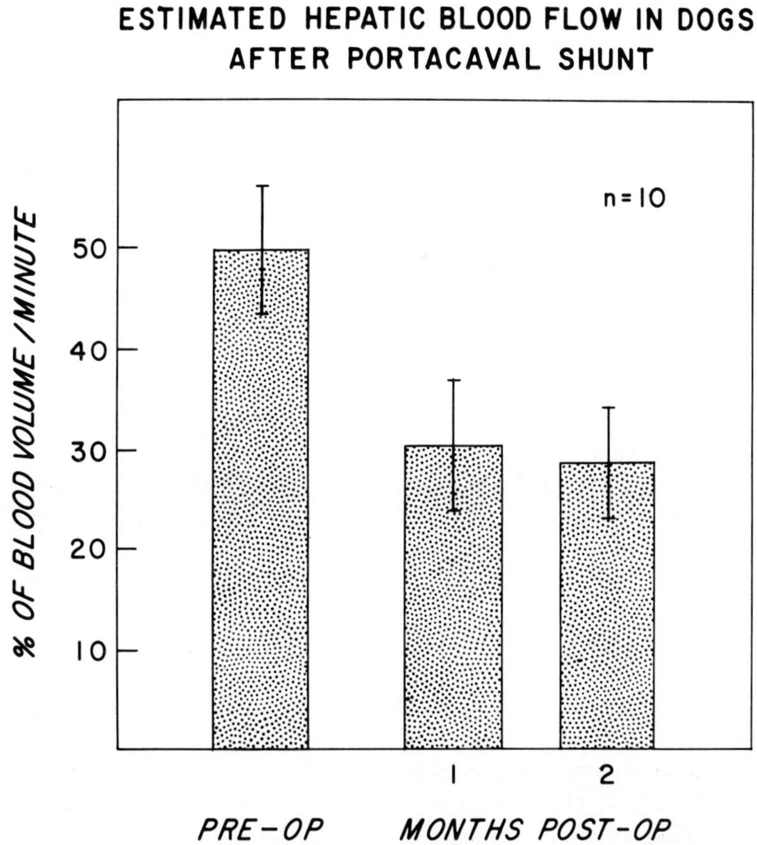

FIG. 3-3. Effect of a portacaval shunt on hepatic blood flow in normal dogs

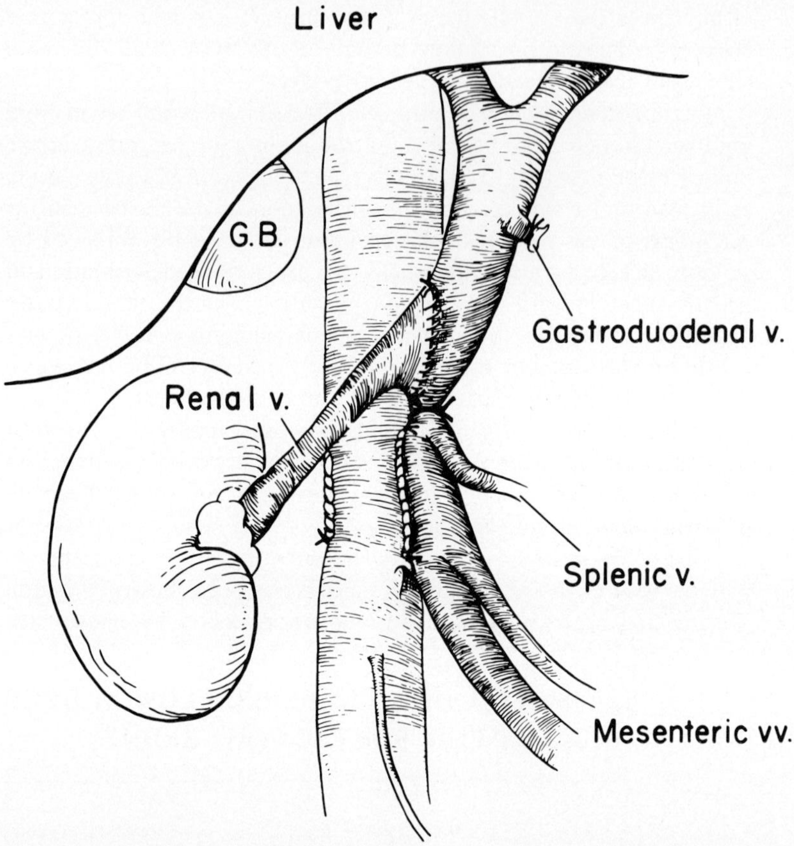

FIG. 3-4. Technique of constructing a renoportal transposition (Reproduced from Ono, H. et. al.: A Technique for Portarenal Transposition in Dogs. Surgery: *63:* 653–657, 1968, with permission of the Publishers)

portacaval shunt in cirrhosis has an unpredictable effect on liver blood flow with some patients showing no significant changes and others a serious decrease. In the groups studied by both Nardi and Warren, the only common denominator of measurements of liver blood flow alone was the fact that those patients who did show significant decrease in flow after shunt had poor results following operation, ranging from early postoperative death with acute liver failure to more chronic problems of encephalopathy and progressive liver failure.

Thus, if one could predict those patients in whom a shunt would result in serious decrease in liver blood flow, better selection and better long term results could be achieved. It is clear that shunts should not be carried out on patients with a normal liver and normal portal circulation, but beyond that, preoperative assessment of liver blood flow alone did not serve as a satisfactory predictor of outcome. At this point, mention should be made of the fact that patients with an extrahepatic block in whom either a splenorenal or a mesocaval shunt is constructed do not show the degree of postoperative complications that besets other groups of patients. Although this has not been

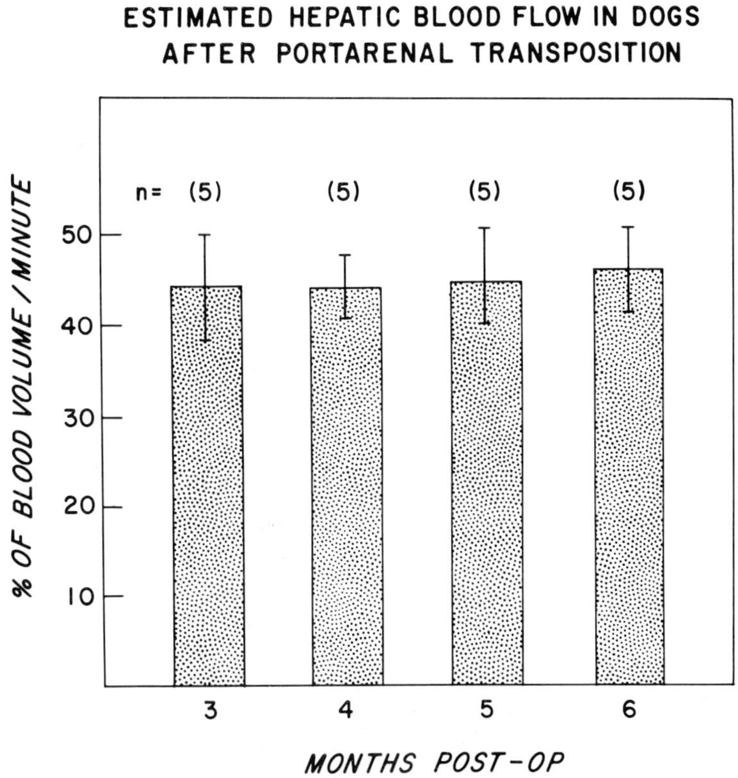

FIG. 3-5. Effect on hepatic blood flow of portarenal transposition

completely explained, the large number of collaterals around the block in the portal vein leading directly to the liver undoubtedly provides for maintenance of portal flow to the hepatic cells, and the distal shunt serves only to decompress the system sufficiently to prevent bleeding but not to bring about serious alterations in the hemodynamics of the liver itself.

pressure changes in portal hypertension

It is generally accepted that portal hypertension is present when levels of free portal pressure over 25 cm. of saline exist in the portal circulation. It is interesting, however, that in patients who have bled from esophageal varices the portal pressure is almost invariably higher than 30 cm., an observation used by Rousselot as a diagnostic tool. By measuring splenic pulp pressure in patients with upper gastrointestinal bleeding in whom esophageal varices are suspected as a source of the hemorrhage, he and his colleagues have been able to discriminate between those patients who are actually hemorrhaging from varices and those who are bleeding from some other source even if they demonstrate changes typical of varices in x-ray films of the lower esophagus. This observation has been confirmed in our own series in which it has been the rare patient who has clearly bled from esophageal varices with a measured portal pressure of less than 30 cm. of saline. In over 90 per cent of elective shunts pressure readings will be between 30 and 40 cm. of saline; in those few instances in which the recorded pressure has been lower than this, there has been some question whether the hemorrhage actually occurred from the varices themselves.

As mentioned above, the change in liver blood flow before and after the construction of a shunt correlates to some degree with the clinical course of the patient and with the occurrence of encephalopathy. Since these observations are of no value as predictors, pressure changes in terms of FPP, HOPP and POPP have been analyzed in terms of the relationship to survival and encephalopathy. In Table 3-1, 83 patients in whom adequate pressure measurements were available have been arbitrarily divided into three groups, depending on the degree of difference between the FPP and HOPP. If the change was negligible (5 cm. of saline) or if there was an increase in HOPP over FPP, there was a death rate during the first year of 19 per cent and a 19 per cent incidence of postshunt encephalopathy. This is in striking contrast to the patients in whom the fall in HOPP was greater than 10 cm. of saline. In this group (corresponding to stage I of Warren's classification), the mortality during the first year after operation was 30 per cent, and 53 per cent of the patients developed recurrent bouts of encephalopathy. If one grades the severity of the encephalopathy, it is obvious that the central nervous system disorder is not only more frequent but more severe. As might be expected, the intermediate group (a drop of 5 to 10 cm.) fell in between the extremes in both mortality and incidence of encephalopathy.

All the cases were graded by the clinical classification of risk described by Child. It is of particular interest that in the stage I cases, 100 per cent of the patients fell in the good to fair category (Child's A and B groups) whereas 24 per cent of the stage III cases fell into the poor risk (Child's C group) category.

Thus, the results described are certainly not caused by a preponderance of poor risk patients in the stage I category. This does

TABLE 3-1. Relationship of Portal Pressure Changes Measured at Operation to Development of Encephalopathy and Late Survival

Difference between FPP and HOPP in Cm. Saline	Total Cases	Postshunt Encephalopathy Grade 1	2	3	4	Total	Category of Risk (Child's Classification) A	B	C	Deaths 3 mos.	3–6 mos.	6–12 mos.	Total (1 year)
>10	17	1	1	4	3	9 (53%)	6 (35%)	11 (64%)	0	4	—	1	5 (30%)
5–10	25	2	4	2	2	10 (40%)	7 (28%)	15 (60%)	3 (12%)	4	1	2	7 (28%)
<5	41	4	1	2	1	8 (19%)	5 (12%)	26 (63%)	10 (24%)	4	1	3	8 (19%)

not imply, however, that clinical evaluation of risk is unimportant since of 13 patients in the entire group who were categorized preoperatively as class C risks, six died within one year of operation and only one patient survived more than nine years.

classification of portal bed block

Traditionally, the classification of portal bed block has been an anatomic one, the cases being divided into suprahepatic, intrahepatic or extrahepatic block. This anatomic division does not, however, help to clarify the pathophysiologic disorders that exist in portal hypertension as much as a newer classification shown in Table 3-2. This involves three general headings, of which only two will be discussed at any length. Cases of portal hypertension caused by a single, large arteriovenous shunt in any of the major branches of the splanchnic, splenic or portal circulation represent interesting but rather esoteric causes of this disease entity; none of them has been studied extensively enough to be analyzed in any detail. Therefore, concentration will be focused on the two divisions of the category referred to as presinusoidal and postsinusoidal portal bed blocks. It should be noted that schistosomiasis and veno-occlusive disease represent almost pure instances of presinusoidal and postsinusoidal block respectively.

Studies on schistosomiasis, therefore, afford an excellent method of analyzing the hemodynamics of presinusoidal block from any cause. In this particular disease in which so-called pipestem fibrosis around the portal triad is the most common hepatic manifestation of the parasitic infestation, von Lichtenberg has demonstrated that, while portal vein and splenic pulp pressures are significantly elevated, wedge

TABLE 3-2. Classification of Portal Hypertension

I. Presinusoidal Block
   A. Extrahepatic (thrombosis of portal vein, occlusion by pancreatic disease, congenital abnormalities)
   B. Intrahepatic
      1. Schistosomiasis
      2. Cirrhosis (primarily periportal fibrosis)
II. Postsinusoidal Block
   A. Suprahepatic (thrombosis or occlusion of hepatic veins or vena cava—Budd-Chiari syndrome)
   B. Intrahepatic
      1. Veno-occlusive disease (Senecio or "bush-tea" poisoning)
      2. Cirrhosis (irregular distribution of architecture with compression or constriction of central veins)
III. Arteriovenous Shunt

and free hepatic vein pressures remain within the normal range, indicating that sinusoidal pressures are also normal. The total hepatic blood flow is normal under these circumstances, and therefore, if the deficit in portal flow exists at all, it is compensated for by an increased flow through the hepatic arterial circulation. This supposition is substantiated by the finding of a decreased oxygen saturation gradient between the hepatic artery and the hepatic vein. Nonetheless, a high degree of prograde flow appears to exist, and portacaval shunts constructed in these patients result in a very striking decrease in liver blood flow and the development of postshunt encephalopathy as well as varying degrees of progressive hepatocellular deterioration.

Similar hemodynamic studies have not been made in cases of veno-occlusive disease (Senecio or "bush-tea" poisoning), but sufficient evidence exists from observations on cirrhotic patients with a high degree of postsinusoidal block, as well as a minority of patients with schistosomiasis in whom disorganization of the hepatic architecture has been demonstrated, to indicate the distinct difference between the presinusoidal and postsinusoidal block. In the latter, *both* the portal vein pressures and hepatic wedge pressures are elevated. Thus, postnecrotic scarring from any cause may lead to impairment of the circulation at the sinusoidal level, the development of a postsinusoidal block and the existence of elevated hepatic vein wedge pressures. In these cases, pressures taken in manometric studies on the portal circulation show that the hepatic occluded portal pressure does not fall significantly and in some instances may actually rise, indicating that the pathophysiologic changes have resulted in the portal vein's functioning as an outflow tract.

In Table 3-2 cirrhosis is classified under both presinusoidal and postsinusoidal block. In the former, one sees minimal disorder of the hepatic lobule and hepatic architecture and very little evidence of cellular necrosis, with the major morphologic change consisting of bands of fibrous tissue surrounding the portal vein. In these cases one finds a normal or only slightly elevated hepatic vein wedge pressure, and measurements in the portal vein at operation show a very significant fall in the hepatic occluded portal pressure. In our own series and in those cases categorized by Warren as stage I portal hypertension, in patients considered to be excellent risks for shunt surgery one finds rather surprising deterioration following the construction of any type of shunt although it would appear that under these circumstances the lesser the shunt (*e.g.,* small splenorenal anastomosis), the less likelihood there is of encephalopathy and deterioration. Conversely, in those patients in whom there is relatively little change in hepatic pressure after portal vein occlusion one finds, as has Warren in his stage III patients, that the construction of any type of shunt that provides combined hepatic or splanchnic decompression (this includes almost any of the commonly constructed shunts except the end-to-side portacaval) is attended by less evidence of postoperative change in liver function and a lesser incidence of encephalopathy. The results of analysis of pressure changes in our own series have been described above and the changes correlated with clinical course and function (see Table 3-1).

Clearly, however, the pathologic changes of all types of cirrhosis are so complex that rarely does one find a case that could be described as a pure presinusoidal or postsinusoidal block. The majority of instances fall on a spectrum between these two extremes, and the pressure studies will vary considerably in terms of the level of hepatic vein wedge pressure and the alteration in hepatic occluded portal pressure following occlusion of the portal vein. Thus, an absolute classification of cirrhosis will not be possible on the basis of either morphologic changes or any of the pressure studies recorded before or during operation. Observations of this type, however, may well lead to a more logical analysis of the hemodynamics.

From the clinical point of view, one usually finds ascites with any high degree of postsinusoidal block except in the rare instances in which there has been significant decompression of the intrahepatic bed by reversal of flow in the portal vein. In these relatively unusual cases the hepatic occluded portal pressure or the portal pressure measured on the hepatic side of the occluded portal vein may actually rise above the free portal pressure, and Warren and others have demonstrated radiographically the reversal of flow in the portal vein under certain circumstances. More reference will be made to the pathophysiology of ascites associated with a postsinusoidal block in a later chapter.

discussion

At the present time a completely logical interpretation of the extremely complex hemodynamics of portal hypertension is not possible, but experimental and clinical studies have led to a physiologic rather than an anatomic classification of the disease and a re-evaluation of the role of shunts in portal decompression. It is clear that a portal-systemic shunt constructed in a patient with a normal liver and portal circulation or in an individual with a nearly pure presinusoidal block will be attended by a serious decrease in liver blood flow, occasionally early postoperative death from liver failure, a high incidence of serious postshunt encephalopathy and the frequent development of progressive deterioration in liver function. In the patient with a nearly pure postsinusoidal block one does not see these postoperative complications if a satisfactory shunt is constructed, such as a side-to-side portacaval shunt, that decompresses both the intrahepatic and the splanchnic circulations. The cases with varying degrees of cirrhosis, which fall between these two extremes on the spectrum, cannot be subjected to such exact evaluation, and selection of the appropriate surgical procedure is not so obvious. Most of these fall into the group categorized by Warren as stage II or intermediate portal hypertension. In general, these patients tolerate portacaval shunt quite well, although further extensive observations and studies will be required to sub-

TABLE 3-3. Concept of Relationship of Pressure Changes to Degree of Cirrhosis and to Postshunt Complications

Stage of Cirrhosis	FPP	HOPP	Wedge Hepatic (Sinusoidal) Pressure	Liver Function	Ascites	Postshunt Encephalopathy	Postshunt Mortality at 1 Year
I (early)	Elevated (>30 cm.)	Less than FPP (>10 cm. difference)	Normal	Good	Usually none	Common and severe	High
II (intermediate)	Elevated (>30 cm.)	Less than FPP	Slightly to moderately elevated	Fair to good	Minimal to moderate	Common but less severe	Moderate
III (advanced)	Elevated (>30 cm.)	Greater, same, or slightly less than FPP (<5 cm. difference)	Elevated	Fair to poor	Moderate to severe	Less frequent and mild	Lowest (<20%)

divide this broad range of hemodynamic changes more accurately and to select therapy more appropriately. From our own data, we would say, however, that patients with a drop in HOPP greater than 10 cm. of saline from the FPP have a diminished chance for survival and an increased incidence of encephalopathy. Presumably (although concomitant flow measurements are *not* available in a significant number of cases), this implies that patients who have significant prograde flow to the liver at the time of shunting will have a greater drop in liver blood flow after shunt and are at more risk of deterioration (Table 3-3).

In an effort to provide a sufficient degree of portal decompression to prevent future hemorrhage but still maintain adequate liver blood flow, both Warren and Britton have described newer types of shunting

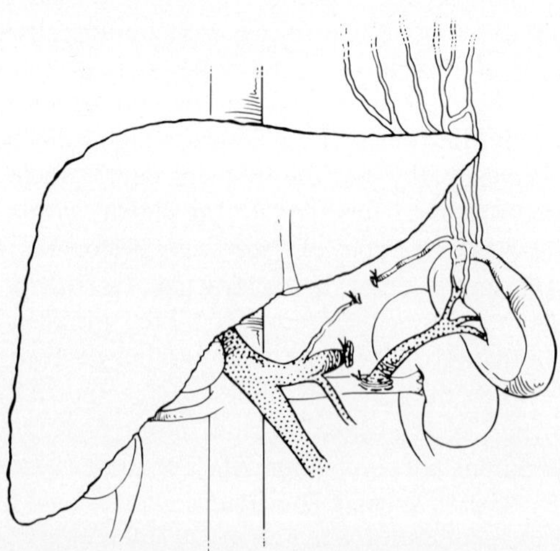

FIG. 3-6. Distal splenorenal shunt (Warren and Zeppa)

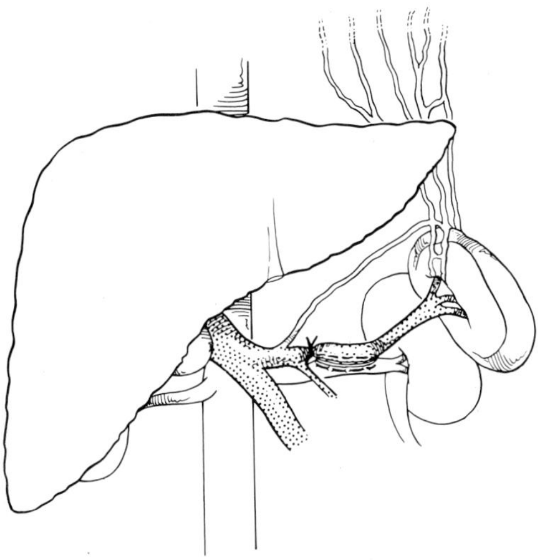

FIG. 3-7. Central splenorenal shunt (Britton)

procedures, which, in their early experience, appear to be associated with much less encephalopathy and liver failure, particularly in patients who might be classified as having a presinusoidal block with the type of hemodynamics described above as occurring with schistosomiasis. These shunts are diagramed in Figures 3-6 and 3-7. In each, the objective is to divert blood away from the esophageal varices without causing a serious degree of diminution in hepatic blood flow. Whether or not these procedures will stand up better than other types of portal azygous disconnections described by Tanner, Allison, Habab and others remains to be seen.

It is certainly in this area of better hemodynamic evaluation of patients with portal hypertension and more appropriate selection of surgical procedures designed to prevent further bleeding that future efforts should be directed. There is considerable hope, however, that with this type of evaluation and approach, some of the serious defects following shunt surgery can be avoided and a more logical approach to the critical problem of bleeding esophageal varices can be achieved.

bibliography

Aldrete, J. S., McIlrath, D. C., and Hallenbeck, G. A.: Effect of portal ligation and of Eck's fistula on hepatic blood flow and concentration of blood ammonia. J. Surg. Res., *7*:504–512, 1967.

Andersen, M. N.: What is "optimum flow rate"? Surgery, *43*:1021–1023, 1958.

Britton, R. C., Voorhees, A. B., Jr., and Price, J. B., Jr.: Perfusion of the liver following side-to-side portacaval shunt. Surgery, *62*:181–188, 1967.

Britton, R. C., Voorhees, A. B., Jr., and Price, J. B., Jr.: Selective portal decompression. Surgery, *67*:104–113, 1970.

Foley, W. J., et al.: Intrahepatic arteriovenous fistulas between the hepatic artery and portal vein. Ann. Surg., *174:*849–855, 1971.

Fomon, J. J., and Warren, W. D.: Rational treatment of gastroesophageal varices. Med. Times, *97:*95–111, 1969.

Gordon, M. J., and Del Guercio, L. R. M.: Late effects of portal systemic shunting procedures on cardiorespiratory dynamics in man. Ann. Surg., *176:*672–679, 1972.

Hassab, M. A.: Gastroesophageal decongestion and splenectomy in the treatment of esophageal varices in bilharzial cirrhosis: Further studies with a report on 355 operations. Surgery, *61:*169–176, 1967.

Hubbard, T. B., Jr.: Carcinoma of the head of the pancreas: Resection of the portal vein and portacaval shunt. Ann. Surg., *147:*935–944, 1958.

Hutchin, P., et al.: Control of portal blood flow—Humoral mechanisms. Ann. Surg., *173:*78–84, 1971.

Kreuzer, W., Schueller, E. F., and Schenk, W. G., Jr.: Hemodynamic studies of cirrhosis in the dog. Surg. Gynec. Obstet., *135:*89–93, 1972.

McDermott, W. V., Jr., and Adams, R. D.: Episodic stupor associated with an Eck fistula in the human with particular reference to the metabolism of ammonia. J. Clin. Invest., *33:*1–9, 1954.

Mulder, D. G., Plested, W. G., III, Hanafee, W. N., and Murray, J. F.: Hepatic circulatory and functional alterations following side-to-side portacaval shunt. Surgery, *59:*923–931, 1966.

Nardi, G. L., McDermott, W. V., Jr., and Dobson, E.: The effect of portacaval shunts on liver blood flow as measured by radioactive colloid. Surg. Forum, *4:*376–380, 1953.

Peters, R. M., and Womack, N. A.: Surgery of vascular distortions in cirrhosis of the liver. Ann. Surg., *154:*432–445, 1961.

Reichle, F. A.: Portal hemodynamics after distal splenorenal (Warren) shunt. Ann. Surg., *176:*195–198, 1972.

Restrepo, J. E., and Warren, W. D.: Liver blood flow after portacaval shunts, hepatic artery ligation and 70 per cent hepatectomy. Ann. Surg., *156:*719–726, 1962.

Salam, A. A., et al.: Hemodynamic contrasts between selective and total portal-systemic decompression. Ann. Surg., *173:*827–844, 1971.

Schenk, W. G., Jr.: Methods for measurement of blood flow. Int. Abstr. Surg., *111:*103–110, 1960.

Smith, G. W., Zug, R. C., and Wilson, S. K.: Periarterial neurectomy of the hepatic artery. An adjunct to portacaval shunt. Amer. J. Surg., *113:*117–123, 1967.

Waddell, W. G., Bouchard, A. G., Wellington, J. L., and Ewing, J. B.: Functional relations of the proximal components of the portal system. A preliminary report. J. Surg. Res., *12:*281–289, 1972.

Warren, W. D., and Muller, W. H., Jr.: A clarification of some hemodynamic changes in cirrhosis and their surgical significance. Ann. Surg., *150:*413–427, 1959.

Warren, W. D., Fomon, J. J., and Zeppa, R.: Further evaluation of selective decompression of varices by distal splenorenal shunt. Ann. Surg., *169:*652–660, 1969.

Warren, W. D., Zeppa, R., and Fomon, J. J.: Selective trans-splenic decompression of gastroesophageal varices by distal splenorenal shunt. Ann. Surg., *166:*437–455, 1967.

Warren, W. D., Fomon, J. J., Viamonte, M., Jr., and Zeppa, R.: Preoperative assessment of portal hypertension. Ann. Surg., *165:*999–1012, 1967.

Warren, W. D., Restrepo, J. E., Respess, J. C. and Muller, W. H., Jr.: The importance of hemodynamic studies in management of portal hypertension. Ann. Surg., *158:*387-404, 1963.

Warren, W. D., et al.: Spontaneous reversal of portal venous blood flow in cirrhosis. Surg. Gynec. Obstet., *126:*315-323, 1968.

Williams, J. H., Jr., and Abelmann, W. H.: Portopulmonary shunts in patients with portal hypertension. J. Lab. Clin. Med., *62:*715-723, 1963.

Witte, C. L., Witte, M. H., and Krone, C. L.: Contrasting hemodynamic patterns of portal hypertension. Ann. Surg., *176:*68-79, 1972.

Womack, N. A., and Peters, R. M.: An investigation of the relationship between portal venous pressure and inferior vena caval and portal venous oxygen saturations. Ann. Surg., *146:*691-699, 1957.

Pathogenesis and Treatment of Hepatic Encephalopathy and the Hepatorenal Syndrome

CHAPTER 4

Until experimental and clinical observations of the past two decades proved to the contrary, the term "hepatic coma" referred to any serious disorder of the central nervous system function associated with liver disease. The presence of jaundice was sometimes related to this ill-defined syndrome, and the word "cholemia" was frequently and vaguely used in clinical parlance. No general recognition was given to the effects of ingested nitrogenous material, and, in fact, a high protein diet was usually urged on patients until they finally slipped into an unresponsive state. Since this effectively prevented protein intake, miraculous if temporary recoveries occurred frequently.

It is always difficult to trace the thread of an idea, but one cannot help but accept the relevance of the remark by Sir Andrew Aguecheek (one of Shakespeare's most confirmed topers), that "I am a great eater of beef, and I believe that does harm to my wit." Regardless of the absolute genesis of the concept, whether from Galen's nebulous concept of humors relating to disposition and temperament or to Shakespeare's astutely phrased observation, it is clear now that "hepatic coma" may be the result of fulminant hepatic disease, chronic and progressive liver failure or the effects of portal-systemic shunting even when there is *minimal* disorder in measurable liver function. A fourth category involves the induction of central nervous system disorders by overly vigorous diuretic therapy or by paracentesis without adequate parenteral replacement. A schematic representation of these patterns of hepatic coma is shown in Figure 4-1.

Although clinical patterns, pathogenesis and etiologic factors may vary, there are certain common denominators in exogenous (portal-systemic encephalopathy) and endogenous (hepatocellular failure) hepatic coma. The electroencephalopathic tracings shown in Figure 4-2 range from normal to the pattern consistent with deep and unresponsive coma. Although similar tracings may be found occasionally in other metabolic disorders, they are so consistent in patients with varying degrees of encephalopathy as to be very helpful in diagnosis and prognosis in terms of response to treatment. Figure 4-3 illustrates the proliferation of protoplasmic astrocytes that is seen in the brains of humans and experimental animals who have died from liver failure or after a series of episodes of postshunt encephalopathy. The distribution of these microscopic changes in the central nervous system varies and to some extent may be correlated with clinical neurologic syndromes. For instance, in a patient whose presenting signs and symptoms of postshunt encephalopathy were those of choreoathetosis, the heaviest concentration of protoplasmic astrocytes was in the basal ganglia rather than in the cerebral cortex.

The problems concerned with ascites will be covered separately, and the end result of progressive hepatic disease is similar in a metabolic sense to fulminant liver failure. Therefore, only two major divisions of hepatic coma will be covered, with the understanding that it is not always possible to draw distinct lines between the clinical syndromes associated with failure of hepatocellular function, the

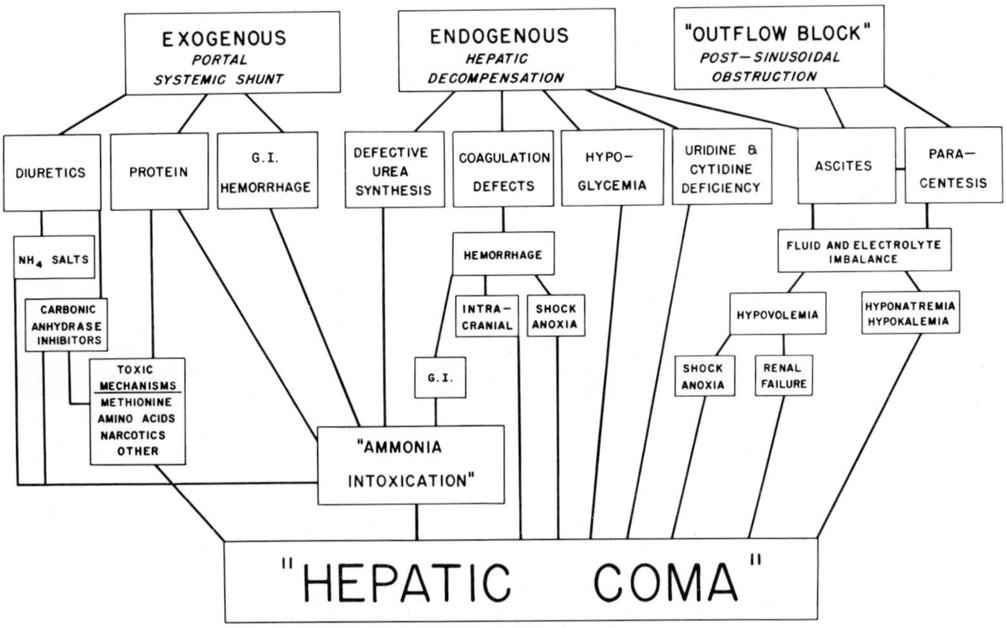

FIG. 4-1. Schematic representation of the patterns of disorders referred to under the vague term "hepatic coma" (Reproduced from McDermott, W. V. Jr.: Postoperative liver failure, Chap. 14, pp. 196–204, in Complications in Surgery and Their Management. Edited by C. P. Artz and J. D. Hardy, W. B. Saunders Co., Philadelphia, 1960, with permission of the Publishers)

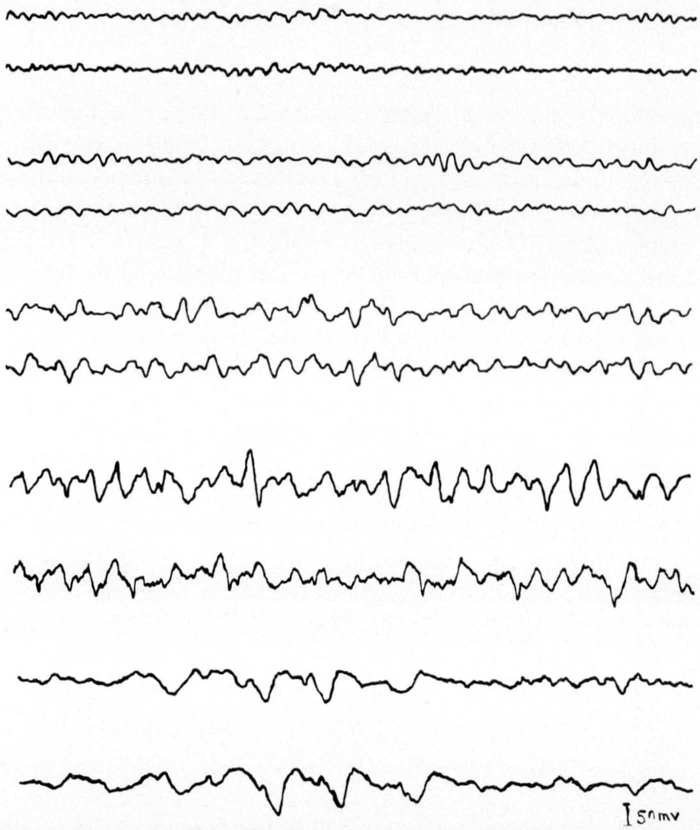

FIG. 4-2. Electroencephalographic tracings representing the changes from normal to those characteristic of increasingly severe hepatic coma

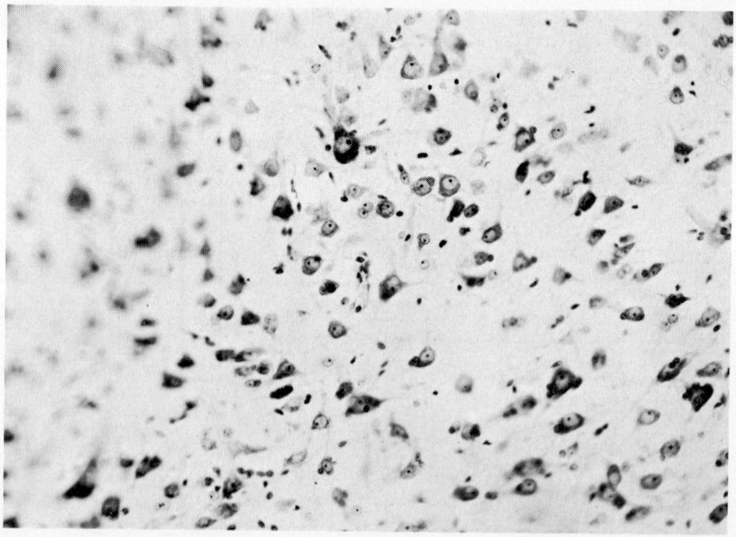

FIG. 4-3. The proliferation of protoplasmic astrocytes in the brain—a microscopic picture characteristically seen in patients who have died while in hepatic coma and in laboratory animals with experimental postshunt encephalopathy

hemodynamic and metabolic changes induced by a portal bed block and the fluid and electrolyte disorders accompanying the accumulation of ascites.

portal-systemic encephalopathy

The central nervous system disorders attendant upon the shunting of portal blood around the liver, and ultimately shown to be intimately associated with ammonia metabolism, have been grouped under the general heading of portal-systemic encephalopathy, exogenous hepatic coma or episodic stupor.

The initial work in this area began in 1877 when Eck illustrated the feasibility of constructing an anastomosis between the portal vein and the inferior vena cava with survival of the animal in apparently good health although with a very short follow-up period. Sixteen years later, during a study of urea synthesis in Pavlov's laboratory, similar animals were prepared. Hahn and his colleagues, working on this problem, observed that these animals manifested a constellation of central nervous system symptoms that the authors related specifically to the ingestion of meat, and since that time, this particular syndrome in the dog has been referred to as "meat intoxication." This syndrome aroused considerable interest over the subsequent decades, but the variability and inconstancy of the symptoms and the inability to define a specific metabolic cause of the syndrome resulted in a confused and confusing picture. Many etiologic factors were suggested including guanidine, amino acids, unknown toxins and bacteriologic and viral infections of the central nervous system. Several observers over the years noted elevation of the peripheral blood ammonia level in these Eck fistula dogs, and Monguio and Krause suggested as long ago as 1934 that this might be the cause of these peculiar symptoms. Since that time the actual existence of the syndrome has been questioned, but studies from our own laboratory in 1954 demonstrated reproducibility of the symptoms and correlation with changes in blood ammonia, provided that forced feedings of meat were given continuously.

Although this syndrome of meat intoxication in the Eck fistula dog was described in 1892, it was not until 1927 that a disorder of ammonia metabolism was suspected by Burchi of causing symptoms in man. Five years later, van Caulert and his associates presented a series of papers that related the ingestion of ammonium chloride by patients with cirrhosis of the liver to subsequent symptoms of drowsiness, confusion and coma.

In 1936, Kirk found elevated levels of ammonia in blood drawn from collateral venous channels in the abdominal wall of a patient with cirrhosis, thus confirming indirectly in man the observations of Folin and Denis in animals that portal blood has a high ammonia concentration.

For over a decade, interest in this phase of liver disease lapsed, and a high protein intake was still considered essential for the recovery of patients with liver disease until several significant reports appeared in the literature. In 1949, Gaustad described a syndrome of "transient hepatargy" in which reversible coma was observed in patients with cirrhosis after gastrointestinal bleeding or the ingestion of protein; he attributed the disorder to absorption from the gastrointestinal tract of the nitrogenous products of enzymatic activity. In 1952 forceful attention to the dangers of ingestion of nitrogenous material by patients with liver disease was drawn by the reports of Gabuzda, Phillips and Davidson and of Phillips and his group in this country and by Stahl and his associates in France. These authors observed that in certain patients with cirrhosis of the liver the ingestion of protein, ammonium salts and ion exchange resins that liberated ammonia produced symptoms of varying severity that resembled the prodromal symptoms of hepatic coma. In the following year, McDermott and Adams reported a case that appeared to correlate the observations on meat intoxication in the Eck fistula dog with the effects of increased nitrogenous intake by patients with cirrhosis. Bizarre episodes of stupor and coma recurred at intervals in a man in whom a direct portacaval shunt was constructed after resection of the portal vein for cancer of the pancreas and in whom ordinary tests of liver function were within normal limits. These episodes were ultimately shown to be associated with the ingestion of protein, urea and ammonium salts. These reversible episodes were correlated with increases in the blood ammonia and with electroencephalographic changes identical to those described by Foley, Watson and Adams in hepatic coma. Thus, it appeared, as Kirk had suggested, that some of the disorders of consciousness in liver disease were caused not by hepatocellular dysfunction but by collateral channels between the portal and systemic circulation. The importance of portal blood bypassing the liver in the presence of intrahepatic block was stressed again by Sherlock and her associates who described several patients with this reversible neurologic disorder and referred to the syndrome as portal-systemic encephalopathy.

It also became apparent that formation and absorption of ammonia from a pool of blood in the colon were major factors in the metabolic and clinical abnormalities seen in patients with bleeding esophageal varices and that correlations could be drawn between blood ammonia levels and the depth and mortality of the associated hepatic coma (Fig. 4-4). The frequency of hyperammoniemia in this group of patients led to the use of ammonia determination in the peripheral blood as indicative that these particular bouts of gastrointestinal hemorrhage were associated with the presence of esophageal varices functioning as portal-systemic shunts. In Figures 4-5 and 4-6, diagrammatic representations are given of the suggested metabolic pathway involved in the production of hepatic coma when excess nitrogenous intake reaches the colon of an individual with portal-systemic shunting.

After these initial reports, considerable attention was focused on this problem. The question obviously arose whether ammonia intoxication was, in fact, a cause of any or all of the clinical cases of hepatic

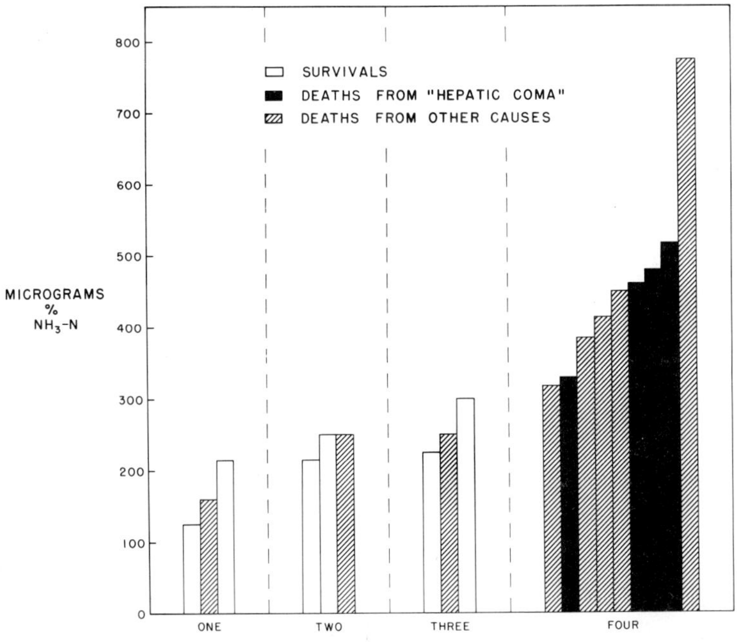

FIG. 4-4. Relationship of blood ammonia levels to the depth of coma and to mortality in a series of patients with bleeding esophageal varices (Reproduced from McDermott, W. V., et al.: Bleeding Varices: A Study of the Cause of the Associated "Hepatic Coma." Ann. Surg. *144*:318–334, 1956, with permission of the Publishers)

coma or whether the elevations in blood ammonia levels in liver disease were similar to the azotemia one finds in renal failure—coincidental with but not a cause of the symptoms. This analogy is unsatisfactory because, unlike the situation in uremia, precoma or coma can be induced by a number of different nitrogenous substances or by certain exchange resins, a common denominator of which is the release of ammonia in the gastrointestinal tract. It is true that the actual level of blood ammonia does not correlate exactly with the patient's clinical state, but if one follows carefully the entire course of a patient with an episode of portal-systemic encephalopathy induced by some type of nitrogenous material in the gut, one finds that the elevation in blood ammonia occurs prior to the appearance of neurologic symptoms. If the source of ammonia production is controlled and eliminated, the ammonia level falls toward the normal range prior to the more gradual recovery of the patient from the episode of stupor or coma. Bessman stressed the importance of arterial-venous differential in ammonia levels of blood taken from the carotid artery and jugular vein; he believed that by this technique cerebral uptake and release can be measured and a more accurate representation of the status of intracellular ammonia metabolism obtained. Summerskill, Wolfe and Davidson amplified these studies and presented a lucid and reasonable explanation of the role of ammonia toxicity in certain types of hepatic coma. Studies by Vanamee and

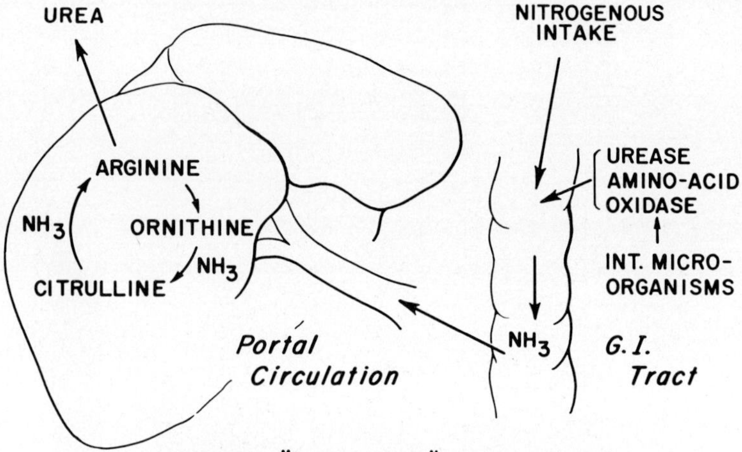

NORMAL " AMMONIA" LEVELS (γ%)

PERIPHERAL	40–70
PORTAL	
Fasting	200–300
After "Nitrogen"	1000–1500
RENAL	
Artery	50
Vein	100

FIG. 4-5. Origin and metabolic pathway of ammonia formed in the colon from ingested nitrogenous material. (Reproduced from McDermott, W. V., Jr.: Progress Reports: Metabolism and Toxicity of Ammonia. N. Eng. J. Med. *257*:1076–1081, 1957, with permission of the Publishers)

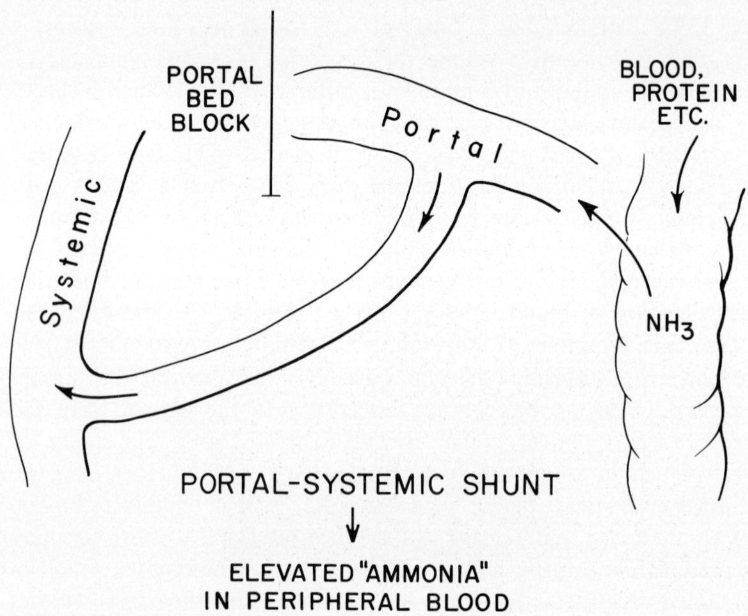

FIG. 4-6. Mechanism by which portal-systemic shunting causes elevations in blood ammonia levels

associates suggested that the additive effect of ammonia-induced respiratory alkalosis was necessary to precipitate overt neurologic symptoms, and other investigators introduced the concept of the partial pressure of ammonia as the important factor in disordered ammonia metabolism and related this to acid-base balance in the body.

management of portal-systemic encephalopathy

After more than a decade of controversy, it is now generally agreed that absorbed ammonia bypassing the liver through surgically constructed or spontaneously developed portal-systemic shunts is a major factor in the central nervous system disorder referred to as hepatic coma or, more accurately, portal-systemic encephalopathy. The mechanism of toxicity is far from clarified, but some evidence indicates that ammonia may interfere with aerobic glycolysis, on which the central nervous system is so dependent, by combining with α-ketoglutaric acid in the Krebs tricarboxylic acid cycle (Fig. 4-7).

More recently, Fischer and his colleagues have published reports on brain amines in acute hepatic coma and on the treatment of hepatic coma and the hepatorenal syndrome with L-dopa and Aramine. They proposed that certain manifestations of hepatic failure might be caused by the accumulation of false neurochemical transmitters that replace the normal transmitters in both the peripheral and central nervous system. Their hypothesis is interesting and is substantiated by a great deal of specific data; it may provide answers to some of the many

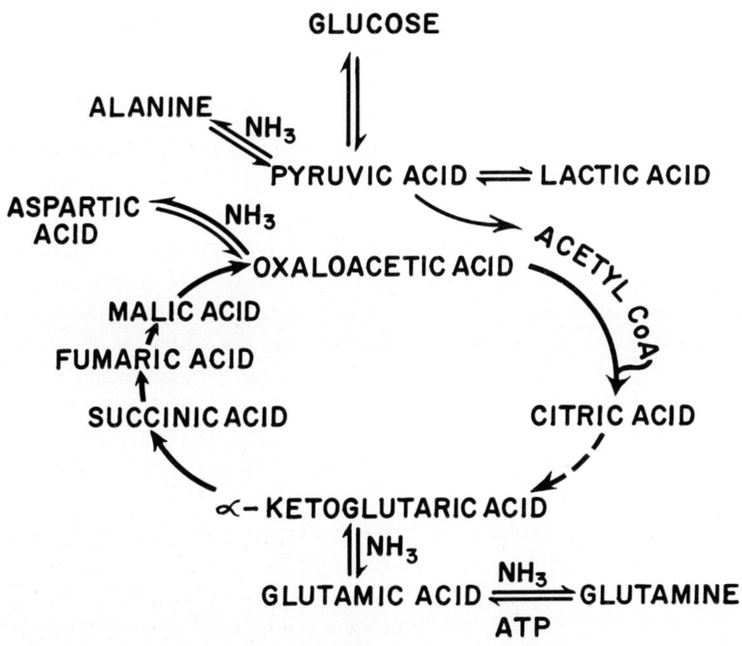

FIG. 4-7. Proposed mechanism whereby elevated levels of blood ammonia may interfere with central nervous system metabolism

unresolved biochemical problems associated with this complicated metabolic disorder. Pursuing their hypothesis still further, Fischer and James have treated several patients with L-dopa and the clinical data were certainly encouraging. In terms of the hepatorenal syndrome, they reported patients treated with metaraminol with apparent diuretic response. The mechanism in this area is less clear even in terms of a hypothesis, but in respect to the concept of false neurotransmitters implementing some of the clinical effects of hepatic failure, the observations are certainly worth further pursuit.

It has also become clear that the varying effects of a shunt on liver blood flow are of great importance as discussed in the chapter on portal hemodynamics. Ammonia clearance after shunting is dependent on normal liver blood flow, and the clinical syndrome of encephalopathy is related to the amount of decrease in total hepatic flow caused by the shunt.

Management of portal-systemic encephalopathy is based primarily on rigorous restriction of nitrogenous material from entrance into the gastrointestinal tract and colon, evacuation of existing material within the colon and alteration of bacterial flora of the colon, all of which are presumptive sources of the enzymatic activity resulting in the formation and absorption of ammonia and other end products of nitrogenous breakdown. In terms of elimination of nitrogenous intake, this implies not only restriction of ingested protein but immediate control of any upper gastrointestinal bleeding, which is, of course, a rich source of breakdown products of nitrogenous material. Cathartics and enemas are used vigorously to empty the colon. Broad spectrum, nonabsorbable antibiotics are effective in altering colon flora and in preventing the formation of ammonia and amines. This concept and method of treatment have been widely accepted, but some recent work by Nance and his colleagues on germ-free animals opened this whole subject to further speculation and study. We have attempted in the past to alter the colon flora by replacement of *Lactobacillus acidophilus,* but, although some success was achieved in a controlled environment, this has not proved practical at the present time in patients outside carefully controlled hospital circumstances. Lactulose, a synthetic disaccharide for which there is no natural enzyme in the gastrointestinal tract, has the effect of lowering the pH in the colon and inducing both an osmotic and an irritative cathartic effect. In our experience, this seemed to be a useful adjunct in the management of patients with chronic recurring encephalopathy, although randomized studies, using sorbitol in the controls, were not conclusive, and approval for general use of this disaccharide is not yet available.

The use of glutamic acid and arginine, both orally and parenterally in soluble forms, has been generally discarded, although at one time enthusiastic clinical reports had appeared in the literature. There is no question that glutamic acid given as a sodium or potassium salt will rapidly reduce the blood ammonia by binding to form glutamine, the level of which rises concomitantly with the fall in ammonia (Figs. 4-8 and 4-9). Arginine, despite apparent clinical effectiveness under

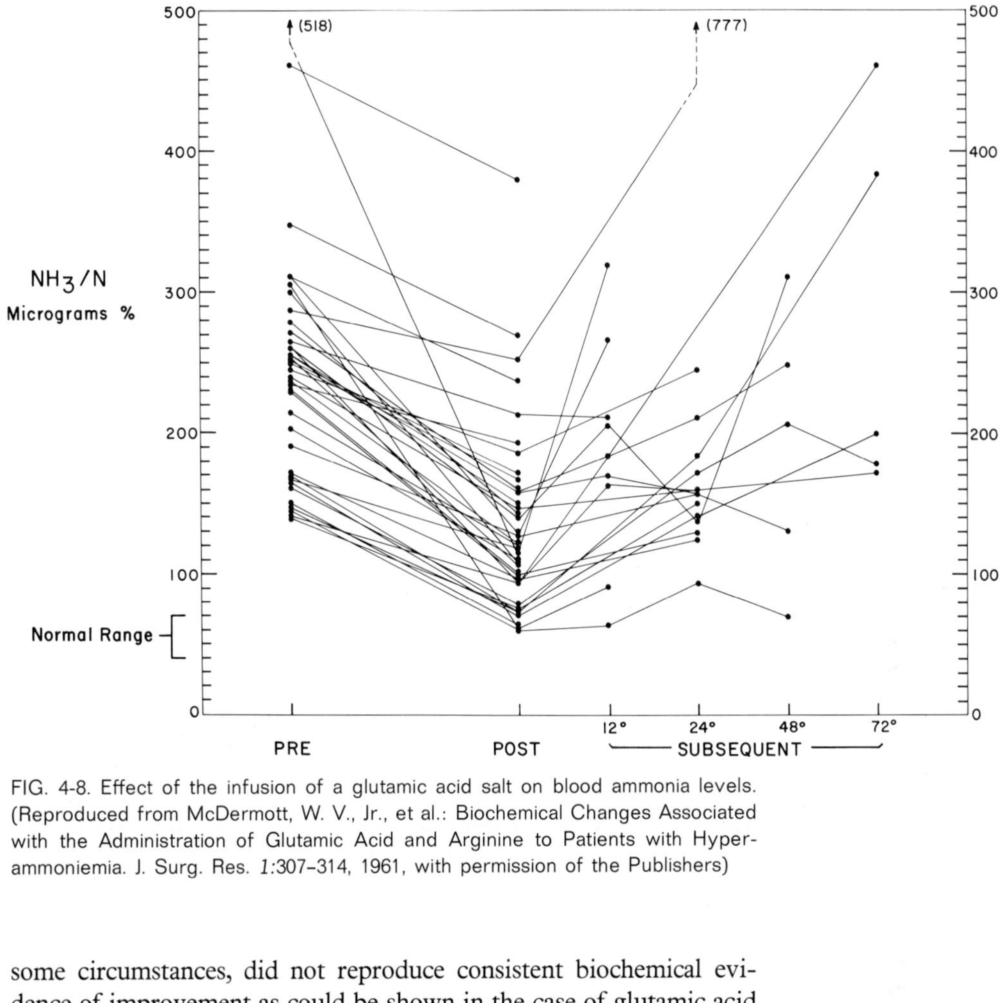

FIG. 4-8. Effect of the infusion of a glutamic acid salt on blood ammonia levels. (Reproduced from McDermott, W. V., Jr., et al.: Biochemical Changes Associated with the Administration of Glutamic Acid and Arginine to Patients with Hyperammoniemia. J. Surg. Res. *1*:307–314, 1961, with permission of the Publishers)

some circumstances, did not reproduce consistent biochemical evidence of improvement as could be shown in the case of glutamic acid (Fig. 4-10). Despite the lowering of the blood ammonia level by administration of glutamic acid, the binding with glutamine is a reversible reaction, and as soon as glutamic acid infusion is stopped, ammonia levels again begin to rise and there is no final clearance from the total body pool, which obviously limits the ultimate effectiveness.

Subtotal colectomy, as reported by Atkinson and Golligher, or surgical exclusion of the colon, as reported by us (Fig. 4-11), does effectively bypass the major source of absorbed materials of nitrogenous breakdown; in selected patients who are refractory to conservative management, striking results have been reported and documented by objective evidence of improvement in the electroencephalogram and ammonia levels (Fig. 4-12). Resnick with the Boston Inter-Hospital Liver Group has reported a randomized study of the effects of colon exclusion in patients with chronic recurring encephalopathy and concluded that this procedure did, in fact, improve protein tolerance, which is the major objective criterion utilized for testing purposes.

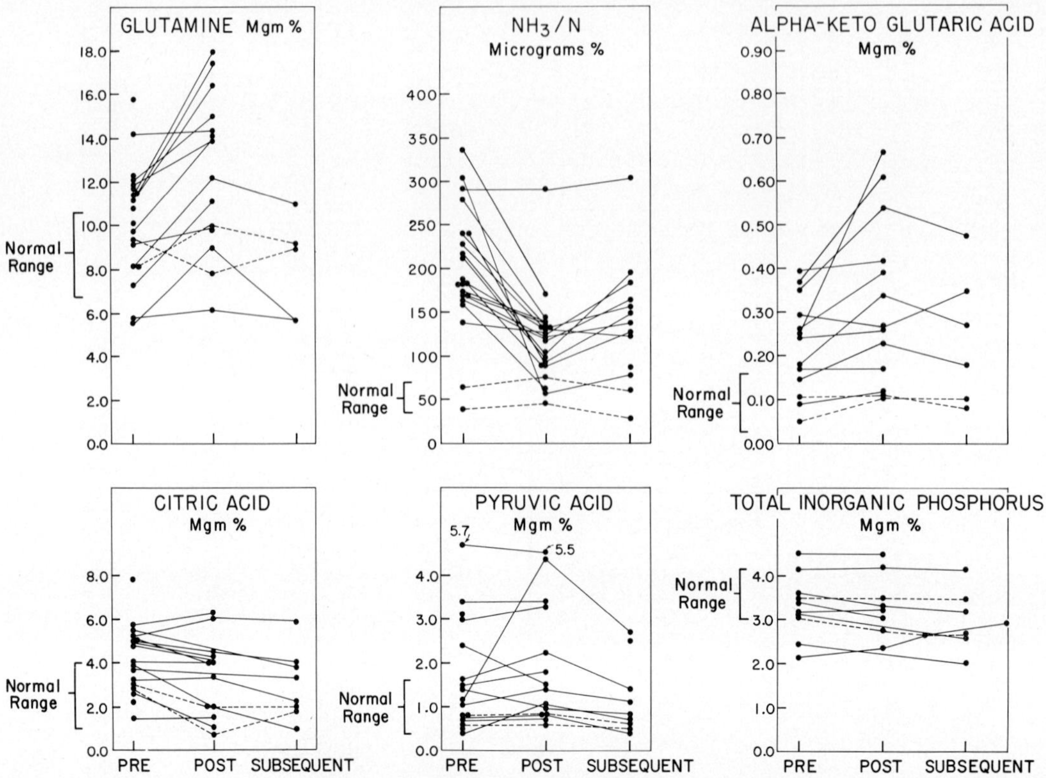

FIG. 4-9. Biochemical changes associated with the infusion of a glutamic acid salt in a series of patients with hyperammoniemia. Dotted lines represent normal individuals. (Reproduced from McDermott, W. V., Jr., et al.: Biochemical Changes Associated with the Administration of Glutamic Acid and Arginine to Patients with Hyperammoniemia. J. Surg. Res. *1*:307–314, 1961, with permission of the Publishers)

More specific information and data on the occurrence of encephalopathy after shunting procedures will be given later in the section on elective portal-systemic shunts and their complications.

fulminant hepatic failure

This syndrome results either from sudden massive liver cell necrosis or from local or systemic stress on an already damaged liver with the sudden onset of terminal liver failure. This, in turn, may result from a severe form of viral hepatitis, as the culmination of extended, continuous ingestion of alcohol ("alcoholic hepatitis"), from traumatic or surgical devascularization of the liver or from the effects of a number of hepatotoxic agents of which halothane has been the most recently described and is, at the present time, the focal point of extensive investigation and controversy. Clinically, the syndrome caused by sudden, widespread dissolution of hepatic cells is manifested by rapidly developing jaundice, lethargy progressing to deep and unresponsive coma, fetor hepaticus and evidence of widespread interference with the clotting mechanism with ecchymosis, nosebleeds, purpura and bleeding from one or more organ systems. Laboratory tests relating to liver function will show bilirubinemia, increase in the alpha amino nitrogen, multiple defects in the clotting mechanism including an increased and fixed prothrombin time unresponsive to parenteral vitamin K administration, and elevations in transaminase levels, which may be extremely high early in the disease but decrease rapidly in the terminal phases when hepatic cell function has almost disappeared.

Although ammonia levels are frequently elevated in patients with acute hepatocellular failure, it is certainly clear that the extremely complex metabolic disorder that occurs with primary liver failure is not explicable on the basis of ammonia intoxication, and, in fact, the extraordinary reserve in urea synthesis permits the clearance of a considerable proportion of the formed ammonia even when many other functions of hepatic cells have deteriorated to extreme degrees.

At autopsy, the liver is shrunken and pale, and microscopic examination reveals ghost cells throughout with little or no evidence of viable hepatic parenchyma. It is a rare but serious disease, and Trey has recorded a fatality rate of 81 per cent in a series of 150 patients who could be categorized as having this form of hepatic coma.

At this point, it is important to expand somewhat on the current

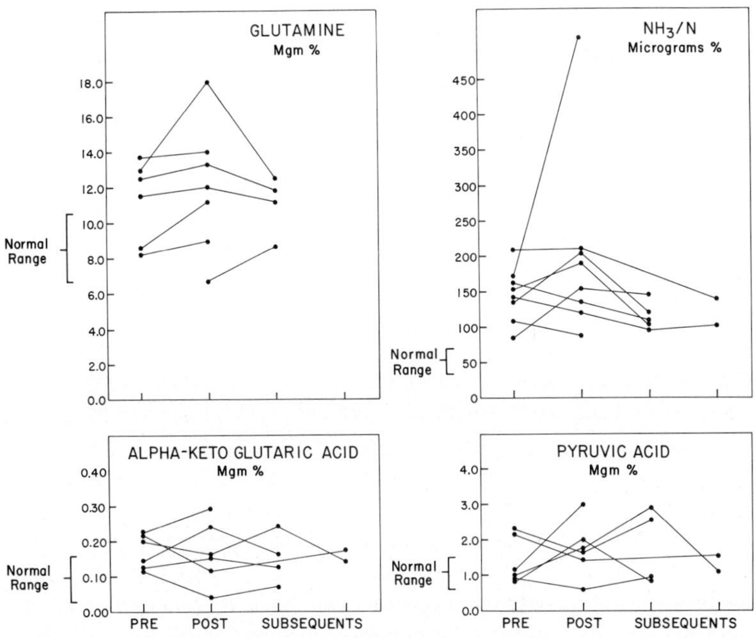

FIG. 4-10. Effects of the infusion of arginine hydrochloride on a series of patients with hyperammoniemia. (Reproduced from McDermott, W. V., Jr., et al.: Biochemical Changes Associated with the Administration of Glutamic Acid and Arginine to Patients with Hyperammoniemia. J. Surg. Res. *1*:307–314, 1961, with permission of the Publishers)

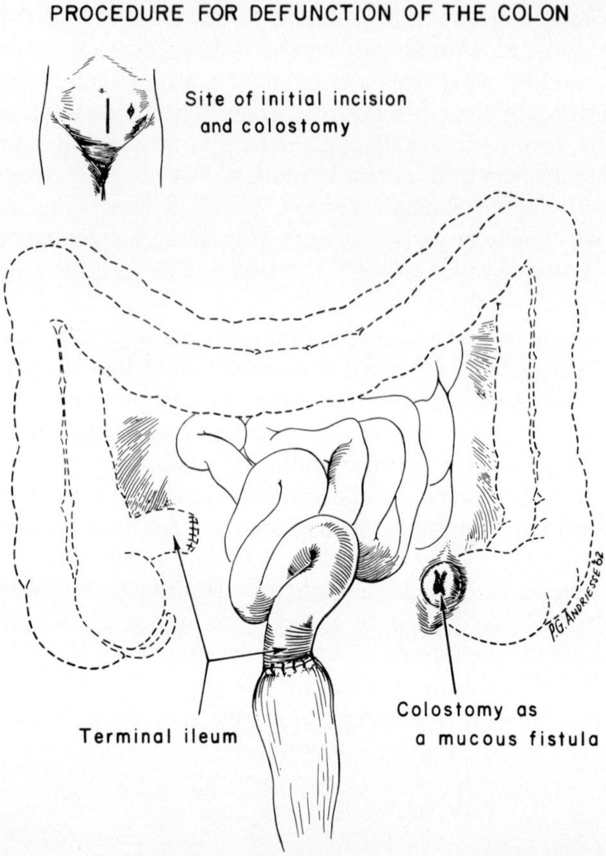

FIG. 4-11. Operative procedure designed to exclude the colon from gastrointestinal continuity as a method of controlling portal-systemic encephalopathy (Reproduced from McDermott, W. V., Jr., et al.: Exclusion of the Colon in the Treatment of Hepatic Encephalopathy. N. Eng. J. Med. *267*:850–854, 1962, with permission of the Publishers)

controversy revolving around the role of halothane anesthesia in the induction of fulminant hepatic failure. Of the patients reported by Trey from the Fulminant Hepatic Failure Surveillance Study, 23 per cent had been exposed to halothane anesthesia within 21 days of the onset of jaundice, and in these, halothane was presumed to be the cause by the reporting physician. Of the 35 patients comprising this group, multiple exposure to halothane within 60 days was noted in 27. Despite the fact that the National Halothane Study did not show any conclusive statistical evidence of hepatic damage related to halothane anesthesia, the increasing number of cases makes it even more likely that diffuse hepatic necrosis may be a rare complication of multiple administrations of halothane. Since the onset of liver failure is not related to the duration of the anesthesia, the severity of the operation or to any factors that might obviously affect the blood supply of the liver, a reasonable working hypothesis at the present time is that some individuals are unpredictably sensitive to halothane or related agents and will respond to the first administration with a rather occult and usually unidentified febrile reaction and then to a subsequent administration with fulminant hepatic necrosis, which has an extremely high mortality rate.

Despite the fatality rate of greater than 81 per cent, even the most apparently lethal clinical syndrome of liver failure may be attended by recovery and ultimate restoration of full liver function. The unpredictable nature of the prognosis makes it difficult to evaluate the various types of treatment that have been employed, but if the full-

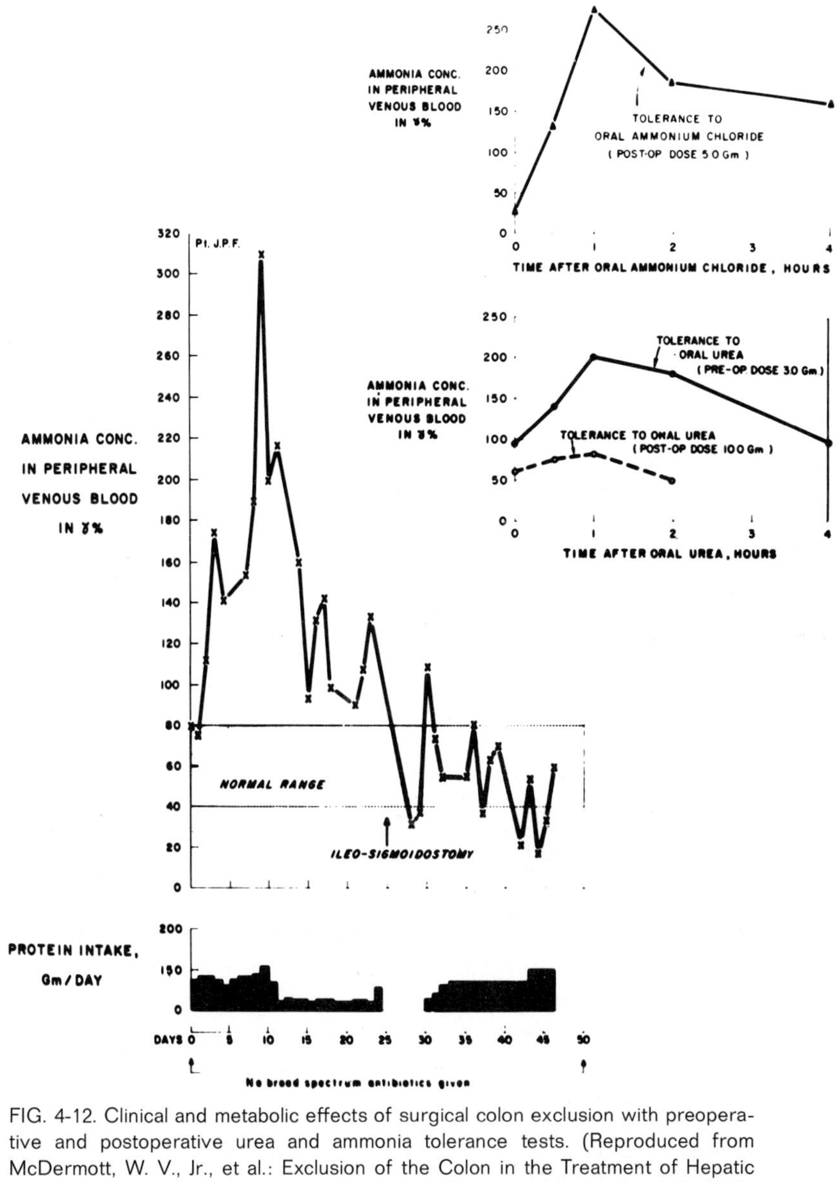

FIG. 4-12. Clinical and metabolic effects of surgical colon exclusion with preoperative and postoperative urea and ammonia tolerance tests. (Reproduced from McDermott, W. V., Jr., et al.: Exclusion of the Colon in the Treatment of Hepatic Encephalopathy. N. Eng. J. Med. *267*:850–854, 1962, with permission of the Publishers)

blown syndrome of hepatic failure is associated with both unresponsiveness and anuria, death has been inevitable in the absence of some form of intervention such as exchange transfusion or auxiliary liver support.

MANAGEMENT OF FULMINANT HEPATIC FAILURE. The management of fulminant hepatic failure is obviously difficult because of the extraordinary number and complexity of the metabolic changes that occur when liver function is suddenly and extremely impaired. Some of the principles used in the management of portal-systemic encephalopathy are also applied to cases of fulminant hepatic failure—restriction of protein, administration of intestinal antibiotics and elimination of all precipitating factors such as sedatives and narcotics, diuretics and local or systemic infections. Complex and multiple disorders of the clotting mechanism are managed in general by the administration of increments of fresh blood or fresh frozen plasma. Since gastrointestinal hemorrhage is an extremely frequent and often terminal complication of severe hepatic failure, vigorous and continuous alkalinization of the stomach has been suggested in order to prevent the multiple superficial gastric erosions that are so frequently a cause of this bleeding. Consumptive coagulopathy is usually a complication of severe infection, and management with heparin introduces another problem in an already extremely complicated program of management. The use of auxiliary liver support by means of perfused calf or pig livers, cross circulation with a human or primate partner or heterotopic transplantation in the experimental animal have all been suggested, studied in the laboratory and used on occasion in the treatment of patients. All of these procedures are complicated, provide only limited and intermittent support, and the overall survival figures have not been encouraging. Repeated exchange transfusions, which were originally suggested by Trey and by Berger, have been widely used and have the advantage of relative simplicity in the management of this extraordinarily complicated problem. It is difficult to gauge the actual effectiveness of this procedure, but individual case experiences have been somewhat encouraging and in a larger series it would appear that an overall increase in survival from 10 to 20 per cent has been achieved.

In our own experience in supporting patients for periods of several weeks with *ex-vivo* pig liver perfusion only to find very little microscopic evidence of regeneration in autopsy studies, it would appear that this highly lethal syndrome could be successfully managed only by long, continuous periods of total hepatic support such as might be achieved by auxiliary transplantation. Further comments on techniques and methods of auxiliary liver support will be provided in a subsequent section.

hepatorenal syndrome

A combination of hepatic and renal failure has long been recognized as a clinical syndrome although it has become increasingly clear

TABLE 4-1. Hepatorenal Syndrome

A. Hypovolemia and prerenal azotemia
   1. Gastrointestinal hemorrhage
   2. Massive and rapid accumulation of ascites
      a. Hepatic failure with postsinusoidal block and hypoalbuminemia
      b. Following paracentesis
      c. Subsequent to end-to-side portacaval shunt (in occasional cases with a high degree of postsinusoidal block)
      d. Gram-negative septicemia
B. Acute tubular necrosis (subsequent to any of the factors above causing renal ischemia)
C. Severe jaundice (usually causing renal failure when associated with depletion of blood or plasma volume)
D. Pre-existing renal disease
E. Other precipitating factors (congestive heart failure, severe pulmonary disease with hypoxia)
F. Dehydration (diuretics, primary water depletion)
G. Hepatic failure (without any of above and without microscopically demonstrable changes in kidneys)—idiopathic

that there are innumerable factors that may come into play in the course of advanced liver disease that may affect renal function adversely. With increasing knowledge of hepatic and renal pathophysiology, groups of patients with both hepatic and renal failure have been identified separately and classified in terms of the precipitating cause of the renal failure. In Table 4-1, an outline is given of the various subdivisions of the so-called hepatorenal syndrome that have been recognized and defined. In any individual case, one or more of these etiologic factors may be present, but there has been increasing recognition that there are a significant number of cases in which oliguria and anuria accompany progressive liver failure without any of the recognized "precipitating factors" and without microscopically demonstrable disease in the kidneys. It is the patients in this latter group who are so puzzling; a number of efforts have been made to establish experimental models in which possible humoral or neurohumoral factors could be studied.

Most of the categories in the table are self-explanatory and need no extensive discussion. *Hypovolemia* from any cause will result in decreased renal perfusion and, with or without liver disease, will cause decreased renal function. Unless a period of renal ischemia ensues, this syndrome is quite reversible, provided replacement with plasma or whole blood, as indicated, is carried out vigorously. If, however, renal ischemia ensues as a result of the decreased renal perfusion, *acute tubular necrosis* may occur and follow a course similar to that seen in patients who develop this lesion without liver disease. Severe and progressive *jaundice* has been implicated both clinically and experimentally with renal failure. It is clear, however, that just the presence of obstructive jaundice alone does not result in severe renal failure, but it would appear from clinical observations and some experimental studies that the presence of deep jaundice in some way sensitizes the kidney to the effects of hypovolemic shock. These conclusions have resulted from studies in pure obstructive jaundice since the frequent presence of jaundice in association with hepatocellular failure introduces the complexities of liver function as well as the effects of bilirubinemia alone. In the presence of *pre-existing renal disease,* it is clearly extremely difficult to evaluate the effects of liver failure, and one must, of necessity, place these patients in a separate category. There are also other precipitating factors such as congestive heart failure with its recognized effects on renal function, any disease process resulting in elevated caval pressure, severe pulmonary disease or other internal or external process resulting in hypoxia, and other more esoteric pathophysiologic disorders, any one of which may of itself interfere with kidney functions. *Dehydration* from any cause will result in decreased urinary output and increased urinary concentration; in association with liver disease, it is usually an excessively vigorous diuretic program that may bring about this result.

When all the patients in whom coexisting hepatic and renal failure are analyzed and classified in a fashion similar to the outline in Table 4-1, there still remains a group of patients in whom the development of severe and progressive renal failure in association with liver failure occurs without any recognizable precipitating factor. It is this group that has particularly puzzled clinicians and stimulated a number of laboratory investigations. Perhaps the most clear-cut evidence that the renal failure is reversible if the liver failure can be controlled comes from the report of transplantation of cadaveric kidneys from patients who died with the so-called hepatorenal syndrome; in this report, a kidney from each of five patients and both kidneys from a sixth patient who died with terminal hepatic and renal failure were transplanted into seven patients with end-stage kidney disease whose liver function was normal. Diuresis and improvement in renal function occurred in all but one recipient; no disease was demonstrated microscopically in any of the transplanted kidneys. In our own experience, several patients with advanced and ultimately lethal hepatic failure had a diuresis and reversal of the biochemical abnormalities associated with oliguria or anuria after *ex-vivo* pig liver perfusion or exchange transfusion. Therefore, although the lethal nature of the hepatorenal syndrome cannot be minimized, it is clear that patients with clinical cases of this dangerous combination may recover without any permanent renal damage and that the transplanted kidney functions immediately upon transfer to a metabolic environment where normal hepatic function exists.

Our own initial studies on a model designed towards experimental clarification of the hepatorenal syndrome seem to indicate that hepatic anoxia resulted in renal dysfunction. Continued studies, however, both on an isolated hepatorenal system and in the intact animal, indicated that crush stimulation of the rich plexus of nerves in the gastrohepatic ligament had a more dramatic and frequently a more permanent effect on renal function than did hepatic ischemia or hepatocellular damage alone. These observations would indicate that a neural or neurohumoral mechanism did exist that would result in both hepatic and renal dysfunction, but it has been difficult to relate these experimental studies to the clinical situations referred to in the discussion above. It is not unlikely that, under certain conditions, severe liver damage results in a metabolic deficiency or in the production of toxic metabolites in such a way that kidney function is affected adversely. Most of the studies available to date would indicate that there is increased renal resistance and decreased renal blood flow in the idiopathic hepatorenal syndrome, but the identification of a deficiency state or a toxic metabolite has not as yet been accomplished. Fischer's concept of the role of false neurotransmitters in the genesis of hepatic coma has also been applied by him in the hepatorenal syndrome, and metaraminol has had a preliminary and limited clinical trial.

Treatment, therefore, is directed toward the correction of any of the possible factors identified in Table 4-1 that might adversely affect renal function and any or all of the mechanisms that may play a role in the syndrome.

bibliography

hepatic encephalopathy

Babior, B. M., and Trey, C.: Drug hepatitis. Int. Anesth. Clin., *8:*329–342, 1970.

Barlyn, L. W., Trey, C., Fagan, J. F., and McDermott, W. V., Jr.: Exchange transfusion for fulminant hepatic failure following hepatic resection. Arch. Surg., *102:*224–226, 1971.

Berger, R. L., and Stohlman, F., Jr.: Evaluation of blood exchange in the treatment of hepatic coma. Amer. J. Surg., *112:*412–418, 1966.

Bessman, S. P., and Bessman, A. N.: The cerebral and peripheral uptake of ammonia in liver disease with an hypothesis for the mechanism of hepatic coma. J. Clin. Invest., *34:*622–628, 1955.

Bessman, S. P., and Bradley, J. E.: Uptake of ammonia by muscle. Its implications in ammoniagenic coma. New Eng. J. Med., *253:*1143–1147, 1955.

Brown, H.: Hepatic Failure. Springfield, Ill.: Charles C Thomas, 1970, 137 pp.

Brown, H., Trey, C., and McDermott, W. V., Jr.: Encephalopathy after portacaval shunting managed with lactulose. Amer. J. Surg., *119:*132–137, 1970.

Brown, H., Trey, C., and McDermott, W. V., Jr.: Lactulose treatment of hepatic encephalopathy in outpatients. Arch. Surg., *102:*25–27, 1971.

Burnell, J. M., et al.: Acute hepatic coma treated by cross-circulation or exchange transfusion. New Eng. J. Med., *276:*935–943, 1967.

Burnell, J. M., et al.: Observations on cross circulation in man. Amer. J. Med., *38:*832–841, 1965.

Clairmont, P., und von Haberer, H.: Ueber Anurie nach Gallensteinoperationen. Mitt. Grenzgeb. Med. Chir., *22:*159–172, 1911.

Conway, E. J., and Cooke, R.: Blood ammonia. Biochem. J., *33:*457–478, 1939.

Davidson, C. S., McDermott, W. V., Jr., and Trey, C.: Sustaining life during fulminant hepatic failure. Ann. Int. Med., *71:*415–418, 1969.

Drapanas, T., et al.: Ammonia intoxication from portal diversion and hepatic failure. Ann. Surg., *142:*560–567, 1955.

Eiseman, B.: Treatment of hepatic coma by extracorporeal liver perfusion. Ann. Roy. Coll. Surg. Eng., *38:*329–348, 1966.

Fischer, J. E., and Baldessarini, R. J.: False neurotransmitters and hepatic failure. Lancet, *2:*75–80, 1971.

Hardison, W. G. M., Greene, E. A., and Norman, J. C.: The viability and effect of flow upon function of the ex vivo perfused pig liver. J. Lab. Clin. Med., *69:*245–255, 1967.

Joyeuse, R., Ivanisevic, B., Longmire, W. P., Jr., and Maloney, J. V., Jr.: The treatment of experimental hepatic coma by parabiotic cross circulation. Surg. Gynec. Obstet., *117:*129–138, 1963.

Kiley, J. E., Pender, J. C., Welch, H. F., and Welch, C. S.: Ammonia intoxication treated by hemodialysis. New Eng. J. Med., *259:*1156–1161, 1958.

Kirk, E.: Amino acid and ammonia metabolism in liver diseases. Acta Med. Scand. (Suppl.), *77:*1–147, 1937.

Kline, D. G., Crook, J. N., and Nance, F. C.: Eck fistula encephalography: Long-term studies in primates. Ann. Surg., *173:*97–103, 1971.

Krebs, R., and Flynn, M.: Treatment of hepatic coma with exchange transfusion and peritoneal dialysis. J. A. M. A., *198:*430–432, 1967.

Lee, C., and Tink, A.: Exchange transfusion in hepatic coma: Report of a case. Med. J. Aust., *1:*40–42, 1958.

Madsen, A. J., et al.: Histamine and mesenteric artery flow in the dog. J. A. M. A., *183:*541–542, 1963.

McDermott, W. V., Jr.: Metabolism and toxicity of ammonia. New Eng. J. Med., *257:*1076–1081, 1957.

McDermott, W. V., Jr., Barnes, B. A., Nardi, G. L., and Ackroyd, F. W.: Postshunt encephalopathy. Surg. Gynec. Obstet., *126:*585–590, 1968.

Mito, M., Pikula, J. V., and McDermott, W. V., Jr.: The effect of portacaval transposition on renal and adrenal function. Surg. Gynec. Obstet., *123:*1289–1296, 1966.

Nance, F. C., and Kline, D. G.: Eck's fistula encephalopathy in germfree dogs. Ann. Surg., *174:*856–862, 1971.

Nienhuis, L. I., Mulmed, E. I., and Kelly, J. W.: Hepatic coma. Treatment emphasizing merit of peritoneal dialysis. Amer. J. Surg., *106:*980–985, 1963.

Onnis, M., Shumacker, H. B., Jr., and Bounous, G.: Blood pressure and renal blood flow response to occlusion of visceral arteries. Ann. Surg., *157:*56–61, 1963.

Ono, H., et al.: Long-term results in portarenal transposition in dogs. Surgery, *64:*214–225, 1968.

Palmerio, C., et al.: Denervation of the abdominal viscera for the treatment of traumatic shock. New Eng. J. Med., *269:*709–716, 1963.

Price, J. B., Jr., Sawada, M., and Voorhees, A. B., Jr.: Clinical significance of intraluminal pH in intestinal ammonia transport. Amer. J. Surg., *119:*595–598, 1970.

Price, J. B., Jr., et al.: Determinants of ammonia tolerance in animals with and without portal systemic shunting. Surgery, *60:*701–709, 1966.

Price, J. B., Jr., et al.: Effects of portal systemic shunting on intestinal absorption in the dog and in man. Surg. Gynec. Obstet., *125:*305–310, 1967.

Price, J. B., Jr., et al.: Mechanism and clinical significance of intestinal ammonia transport. Surg. Forum, *18:*331–333, 1967.

Raskin, N. H., Price, J. B., Jr., and Fishman, R. A.: Portal-systemic encephalopathy due to congenital intrahepatic shunts. New Eng. J. Med., *270:* 225–229, 1964.

Resnick, R. H., et al.: A controlled trial of colon bypass in chronic hepatic encephalopathy. Gastroenterology, *54:*1057–1069, 1968.

Saravis, C. A., Trey, C., and Grady, G. F.: Rapid screening test for detecting hepatitis-associated antigen. Science, *169:*298–299, 1970.

Stahl, J.: Studies of the blood ammonia in liver disease. Its diagnostic, prognostic, and therapeutic significance. Ann. Int. Med., *58:*1–24, 1963.

Storb, R., et al.: Clinical and hematologic effects of cross circulation in baboons. Transfusion, *9:*23–31, 1969.

Subcommittee on the National Halothane Study of the Committee on Anesthesia, National Academy of Sciences-National Research Council: Summary of the National Halothane Study. Possible association between halothane anesthesia and postoperative hepatic necrosis. J. A. M. A., *197:*775–788, 1966.

Trey, C.: The critically ill child: Acute hepatic failure. Pediatrics, *45:*93–98, 1970.

Trey, C., and Davidson, C. S.: The management of fulminant hepatic failure. Progr. Liver Dis. *3:*282–298, 1970.

Trey, C., Burns, D. G., and Saunders, S. J.: Treatment of hepatic coma by exchange blood transfusion. New Eng. J. Med. *274:*473–481, 1966.

Trey, C., Lipworth, L., and Davidson, C. S.: The clinical syndrome of halothane hepatitis. Anesth. Analg. (Cleveland) *48:*1033–1042, 1969.

Trey, C., Brown, H., Goransky, L., and McDermott, W. V., Jr.: Lactulose treatment of hepatic encephalopathy: Effects on carbohydrate metabolism and colonic hydrogen ion concentration. Surg. Forum, *21:*355–356, 1970.

Trey, C., et al.: Massive liver necrosis in the monkey: The effects of exchange blood transfusions on fulminant liver failure. J. Lab. Clin. Med. *73:* 784–794, 1969.

Trey, C., et al.: Fulminant hepatic failure. Presumable contribution of halothane. New Eng. J. Med., *279:*798–801, 1968.

Voorhees, A. B., Jr., and Price, J. B., Jr.: Surgical treatment of hepatic encephalopathy. Ann. N.Y. Acad. Sci., *170:*259–266, 1970.

Walshe, J. M.: Hepatic coma. Postgrad. Med. J., *32:*467–472, 1956.

Whitcomb, F. F., Trey, C., and Braasch, J. W.: Preoperative preparation of the jaundiced patient. A review of current practice. Surg. Clin. N. Amer., *50:*663–682, 1970.

Wilson, R. D., Tarrow, A. B., and Garvin, S.: Hepatic effects of halothane: A clinical and laboratory evaluation of 10,129 administrations. Anesth. Analg. (Cleveland), *43:*40–43, 1964.

Zuidema, G. D., et al.: Blood ammonia studies in monkeys before and after portacaval anastomosis. Arch. Surg., *85:*152–157, 1962.

hepatorenal syndrome

Dawson, J. L.: Jaundice and anoxic renal damage: Protective effect of mannitol. Brit. Med. J., *1:*810, 1964.

Dawson, J. L.: Post-operative renal function in obstructive jaundice: Effect of a mannitol diuresis. Brit. Med. J., *1:*82–86, 1965a.

Dawson, J. L.: The incidence of postoperative renal failure in obstructive jaundice. Brit. J. Surg., *52:*663–665, 1965b.

Dawson, J. L.: Acute post-operative renal failure in obstructive jaundice. Ann. Roy. Coll. Surg. Eng., *42:*163–181, 1968.

Editorial: Renal abnormalities in Laennec's cirrhosis. J. A. M. A., *181:*990–991, 1962.

Fischer, J. E., and Baldessarini, R. J.: Renal changes in hepatic failure. Lancet, *2:*769–770, 1971.

Fischer, J. E., and James, J. H.: Treatment of hepatic coma and hepatorenal syndrome. Mechanism of action of L-dopa and aramine. Amer. J. Surg., *123:*222–230, 1972.

Garrett, J. C., Voorhees, A. B., Jr., and Sommers, S. C.: Renal failure following portasystemic shunt in patients with cirrhosis of the liver. Ann. Surg., *172:*218–225, 1970.

Gliedman, M. L., Carroll, H. J., Popowitz, L., and Mullane, J. F.: An experimental hepatorenal syndrome. Surg. Gynec. Obstet., *131:*34–40, 1970.

Goldstein, H., and Boyle, J. D.: Spontaneous recovery from the hepatorenal syndrome. Report of four cases. New Eng. J. Med., *272:*895–898, 1965.

Hori, M., Austen, W. G., and McDermott, W. V., Jr.: Hepatic anoxia and stimulation of hepatic nerves on renal hemodynamics and function. Surg. Forum, *15:*108–109, 1964.

Hori, M., Austen, W. G., and McDermott, W. V., Jr.: Role of hepatic arterial blood flow and hepatic nerves on renal circulation and function: I. Acute studies in the dog. Ann. Surg., *162:*849–862, 1965a.

Hori, M., Austen, W. G., and McDermott, W. V., Jr.: Role of hepatic arterial blood flow and hepatic nerves on renal circulation and function: II. Chronic studies in the dog. Ann. Surg., *162:*949–958, 1965b.

Hori, M., Neto, A. C., Austen, W. G. and McDermott, W. V., Jr.: Isolated in vivo hepatorenal perfusion in the dog. Circulatory and functional response of the kidney to hepatic anoxia. J. Surg. Res. *7:*413–417, 1967.

Hori, M., et al.: Nerve influence on the splanchnic circulation. Recent Advances Gastroent., *2:*581–584, 1966.

Koppel, M. H., et al.: Transplantation of cadaveric kidneys from patients with hepatorenal syndrome. Evidence for the functional nature of renal failure in advanced liver disease. New Eng. J. Med., *280:*1367–1371, 1969.

Liebowitz, H. R.: Primary kidney disease in patients with cirrhosis of the liver. New York J. Med., *65:*535–541, 1965.

Mashford, M. L., Mahon, W. A., and Chalmers, T. C.: Studies of the cardiovascular system in the hypotension of liver failure. New Eng. J. Med., *267:*1071–1074, 1962.

Papper, S., Belsky, J. L., and Bleifer, K. H.: Renal failure in Laennec's cirrhosis of the liver. I. Description of clinical and laboratory features. Ann. Int. Med., *51:*759–773, 1959.

Resnick, R. H., Chalmers, T. C., Chatterjee, G. P., and Madoff, M. M.: Renal function and fecal flora after colon bypass. Arch. Surg., *101:*353–358, 1970.

Summerskill, W. H. J.: Hepatic failure and the kidney. Gastroenterology, *51:*94–107, 1966.

Thompson, E. N., Cawdery, J., and Martin, J.: Hepatic coma with renal failure, treated by repeated exchange transfusion. Arch. Dis. Child., *43:*368–371, 1968.

Topuzlu, C., and Stahl, W. M.: Effect of bile infusion on the dog kidney. New Eng. J. Med., *274:*760–763, 1966.

Pathogenesis and Treatment of Cirrhotic Ascites

CHAPTER 5

The term ascites, which, from its Greek derivation, refers to a bag of fluid, is used in medical terminology to refer to any collection of fluid within the peritoneal cavity. There are a number of different causes for the accumulation of ascitic fluid, and one must establish some type of categorization in order to present a comprehensible discussion. It has been customary to classify ascites under two major headings: exudative and transudative, terms which in a broad sense are self-explanatory. Since we are primarily concerned with the liver, only a few introductory comments will be made relative to the disease processes classified under *exudative ascites.* This term refers, in general, to the accumulation of peritoneal fluid that results from an excess outpouring of liquid of high specific gravity and high protein content from either an inflammatory or neoplastic process within the abdominal cavity. Since there is a free exchange between the peritoneal cavity and the vascular compartment, the exudation of fluid must be in excess of the resorbing capacity of the serous lining of the abdomen. In a process of equilibration under these circumstances, the ascitic fluid is more likely to draw water from the intravascular compartment because of its high protein content than it is to be resorbed.

In Table 5-1 a simplified categorization of the various causes for the accumulation of ascitic fluid is given and the distinctions drawn primarily on the level of protein content, which is usually greater than 3.0 gm. per 100 ml. in exudative ascites and less than this in transudative ascites.

Among the different causes of exudative ascites, the one that is most likely to cause confusion in relation to cirrhosis is the relatively rare syndrome referred to as pancreatic ascites. Occasionally, following trauma or inflammation, the rupture of the pancreatic ductile

TABLE 5-1. Ascitic Fluid

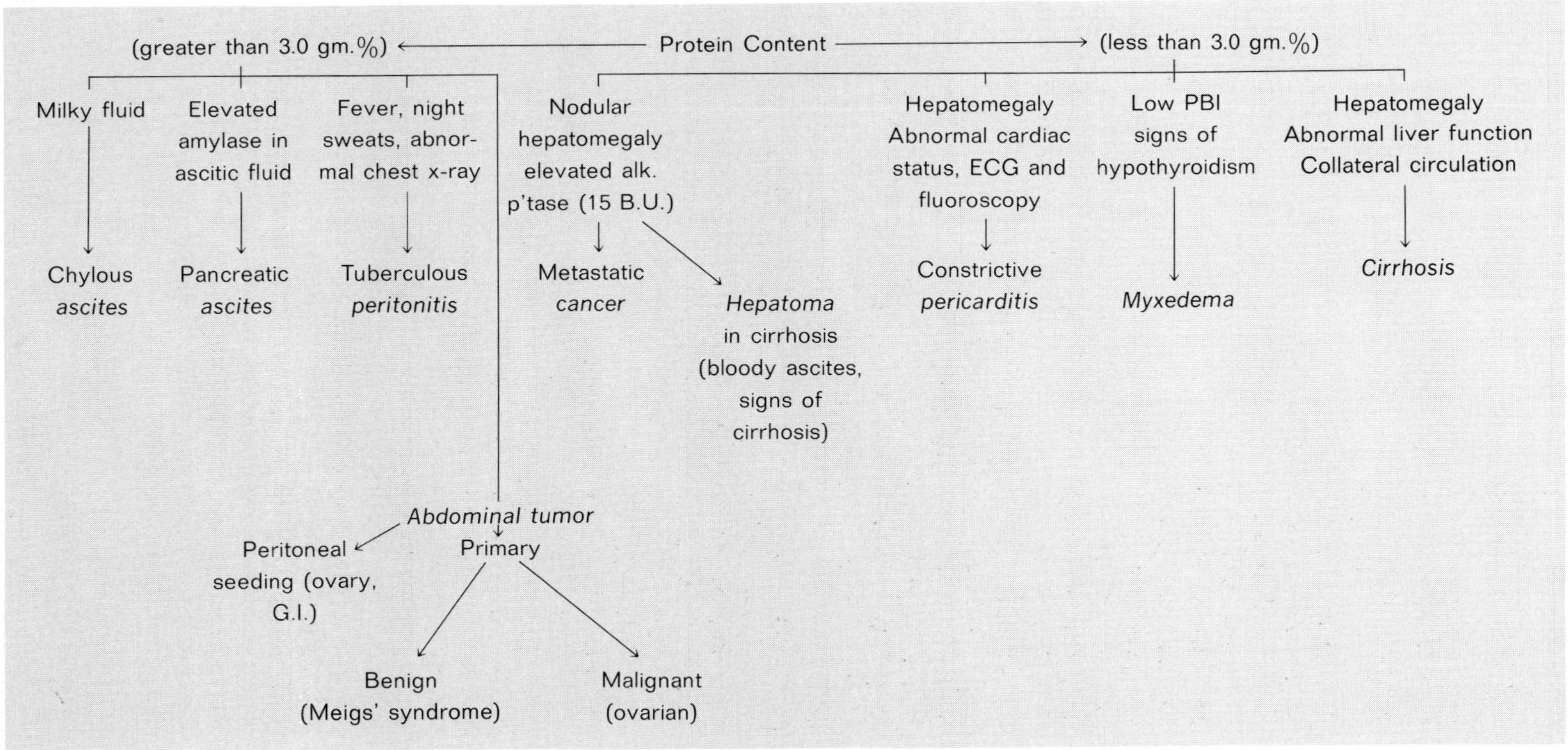

system results in the establishment of a communication with the free peritoneal cavity rather than a localized inflammatory mass or pseudocyst. Since many of the patients with pancreatitis are chronic alcoholics, accumulation of fluid under these circumstances and without signs of inflammation may easily lead to confusion in the actual diagnosis. If one considers the possibility of pancreatic ascites, the syndrome is distinctive—the peritoneal fluid has a high specific gravity, high protein content, and very high amylase level, and the serum amylase level is usually although not invariably elevated.

It is with the general phenomenon of *transudative ascites* and more specifically cirrhotic ascites that we will be primarily concerned. The accumulation of fluid within the peritoneal cavity in this type is secondary to transudation from capillary or sinusoidal beds and from the lymphatics of the splanchnic and hepatic circulations. This, in turn, may be caused by increased venous pressure secondary to a number of disorders. Obstruction of the hepatic venous outflow either from thrombosis or abnormalities in the development of the inferior vena cava or hepatic venous circulation or from the retrohepatic extension of malignant disease causes intractable ascites and is referred to as the Budd-Chiari syndrome.

Fibrous obstruction of the inferior vena cava above the liver with intractable ascites was first reported by Osler in 1878. Since then, 17 similar cases of stricture by either fibrosis or a congenital web have been reported, and this total experience has been reviewed and summarized in an article by Schaffner and associates. Although the disease is presumably congenital in origin, the symptoms generally begin in early adult life and have persisted as long as 20 years. Definition of the lesion can be accomplished by catheterization studies of the vena cava with angiography. Recognition of this syndrome is particularly important since the lesion is usually correctable by one of a variety of surgical procedures.

Disease within the liver itself (usually caused by cirrhosis but rarely by an interesting and bizarre entity known as bush-tea poisoning) may be associated with the formation of ascites. Congestive heart failure may result not only in the accumulation of abdominal fluid but also in the development of a type of cirrhotic process; a discussion of the physiologic derangements and treatment of this disorder is, however, beyond the defined scope of this review. Hence, our attention will be focused primarily on the problems of accumulated ascitic fluid secondary to cirrhosis of the liver.

A discussion of the pathophysiology of ascites in hepatic disease should be prefaced by a review of the methods by which ascites can be produced in the experimental animal in order to provide a proper framework for the understanding of the complicated sequence of events that occurs clinically.

experimental production of ascites

Almost 300 years ago Richard Lower of London recorded that ligation of the thoracic inferior vena cava of the dog resulted consistently in the development of ascitic fluid. Based on these perceptive observations, constriction of the suprahepatic vena cava was for years the standard laboratory technique for inducing and studying the formation of ascites. Subsequently, this laboratory technique has been refined by Orloff and others to a method by which selective ligation of the majority of the hepatic veins and partial compression by a choker of the remaining venous outflow from the liver can be used to produce a controlled experimental situation. It was recognized long ago that while occlusion or constriction of the outflow from the liver consistently resulted in the formation of ascitic fluid, portal vein obstruction did not. Even if hypoproteinemia is induced by repeated plasmaphereses in association with portal vein constriction, the ascites that does form has a very low protein content and differs considerably from the ascites seen in man, which is more comparable to the fluid that develops after an outflow block.

the pathogenesis of cirrhotic ascites

The mechanisms involved in the formation of cirrhotic ascites are still somewhat confusing because the complex hemodynamic and metabolic changes that occur have not yet been fully clarified. By piecing together the experimental and clinical evidence available, however, one can develop a clearer picture of the disordered pathophysiology than was possible even a few years ago. A number of specific facts and observations are particularly significant: (1) Ascitic fluid has approximately the same composition as liver lymph; the lymphatics in the liver hilus and gastrohepatic ligament are greatly increased in size and number, and in experimental studies transudation from these lymphatics and from the liver itself accounts for a major portion of the accumulated intraperitoneal fluid. (2) The experimental production of ascites can be easily accomplished by any procedure that obstructs the outflow from the liver but not by obstruction of the portal vein itself unless, as described above, hypoproteinemia is induced. (3) The increased intrahepatic portal pressure seen in cirrhosis with ascites does not fall within the normal range after occlusion of the portal vein, and further decrease requires obstruction of the hepatic arterial inflow; presumably this is on the basis of intrahepatic arterial-portal shunts and is seen with cirrhosis but not in the normal individual or laboratory animal. (4) In cirrhotic ascites there is abnormal retention of water and sodium; restriction of salt alone may bring about an amelioration or dissipation of the accumulated fluid. (5) Increased aldosterone activity is a consistent pattern, and it is probable that the increased aldosterone levels are related not to failure of detoxification by the damaged liver but rather to the effect on volume receptors of a decreased effective circulating blood volume; other mechanisms such as hypokalemia may also be related to the induction of aldosterone secretion from the adrenal. (6) The serum albumin level and, therefore, the intravascular osmotic pressure are usually decreased.

While there are admittedly many factors involved in the formation of cirrhotic ascites, certainly an alteration in the normal hemodynamics of the liver plays a major role, and an intrahepatic postsinusoidal outflow block is undoubtedly a very important factor in the ascites seen with various forms of liver disease. While the morphologic and hemodynamic changes found in association with cirrhosis vary widely, certain observations have been generally accepted. These tend to support the fact that postsinusoidal block of varying degree does exist in many types of liver disease and that shunts between the arterial and portal circulations within the liver do exist as a part of the general pattern. It is difficult to relate these changes specifically to the degree and relative intractability of ascites because a postsinusoidal block is not the sole factor contributing to the retention of intraperitoneal fluid with liver disease. The fall in intravascular osmotic pressure from depressed serum albumin levels certainly is important since the integrity of the vascular compartment is maintained primarily by the circulating plasma proteins. Although equilibration of intravenously administered albumin between the vascular and interstitial compartments occurs rapidly, normally the plasma proteins that leak from the proximal end of the capillary or sinusoidal bed are returned to the blood so that osmotic equilibrium remains undisturbed. With cirrhotic ascites, one frequently finds a combination of depression in serum albumin and a resulting drop in osmotic pressure together with the increased pressure at the distal end of the capillary or sinusoidal bed.

One must also consider the role of endocrine factors and the alteration of renal function that occurs in the presence of ascites and, most important, delineation of the part played by increased circulating levels of aldosterone in the abnormal retention of sodium and water that has been referred to above. Increased secretion of antidiuretic hormone may be an accessory endocrine factor in the syndrome but probably does not play a role comparable to that of aldosterone. The characteristic change in renal function that occurs is a voracious retention of sodium by the kidney with an increased excretion of potassium in the urine. Thus, in most of the patients with relatively intractable ascites, one would find less than 5 mEq. per L. of sodium in the urine, in contrast to the increased excretion of potassium, which may be two or three times the normal amount.

In summary, one could say that the accumulation of ascitic fluid in connection with cirrhosis is caused in part by the development of a postsinusoidal block in association with a depression of serum albumin and a resulting decrease in osmotic pressure. The endocrine changes are probably secondary manifestations of changes in plasma volume, osmolarity, hypokalemia and hepatic blood flow. A simplified diagram of the pathogenesis of cirrhotic ascites is given in Figure 5-1.

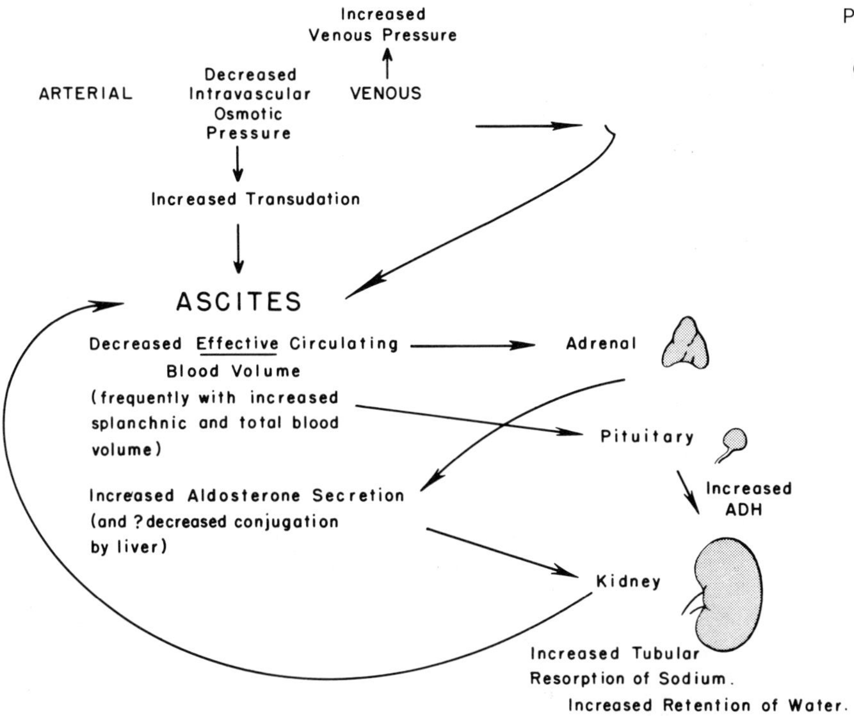

FIG. 5-1. Pathogenesis of ascites: splanchnic and intrahepatic portal vascular beds

treatment of ascites

medical

The patient with cirrhotic ascites will present primarily as a problem in medical management, but the surgeon is frequently involved in the problem if the ascites proves to be refractory because of a high degree of outflow block or if there is associated bleeding from esophageal varices that requires surgical intervention before a desirable period of a diuretic program can be completed. As described above, the appearance of ascites is determined primarily by two factors, the falling serum albumin level and the increased intrahepatic portal venous pressure. The rate at which ascitic fluid accumulates, however, is a reflection of the disparity between dietary sodium intake and sodium excretion; an understanding of sodium balance is certainly the keystone of successful management.

Under ordinary conditions of external environment, an afebrile patient will rarely excrete more than 10 mEq. daily in the sweat. The major route of sodium excretion is the kidney, and under normal circumstances, an individual with an intake of 5 to 8 gm. of salt daily will show urinary excretion of 80 to 100 mEq. per L. of sodium in the urine with concomitant potassium excretion in the range of 40 to 50 mEq. per L. With accumulating or refractory cirrhotic ascites, however, the situation is drastically altered, and there may be sodium excretion in the urine of 0 to 5 mEq. per L. because of the voracious retention of sodium by the kidney. Therefore, in a patient who may be excreting only 15 to 20 mEq. of sodium daily in both the urine and the sweat, a dietary intake as low as 1 gm. daily will still result in a net daily increase in the total body sodium and concomitant retention of water, both of which are reflected primarily in a progressive increase in the ascites. Treatment must therefore focus on both rigid restriction of the sodium intake (a diet with less than 200 mg. of salt daily can be contrived) and efforts to increase the loss of sodium through the kidney.

The introduction of the chlorothiazide drugs, which effectively increase the excretion of sodium by the kidney, proved to be a major advance in satisfactory medical management of ascites. Shortly after they were utilized widely, it became apparent that their use was frequently attended by a form of hepatic encephalopathy or coma. Despite extensive studies on this phenomenon, it is still not clear whether the central nervous system disorder is caused by the recognized losses of potassium in the urine and the concomitant hypokalemia, by the increased production of ammonia by the kidney or by some other as yet undefined metabolic disorder. At any rate, the use of a greatly increased intake of potassium in association with chlorothiazide administration appears to have limited the risks associated with the use of these drugs.

When the importance of hyperaldosteronism in this syndrome was recognized, pharmacologic agents designed to counteract the effect of aldosterone were introduced. Treatment with spironolactones as aldosterone antagonists was followed by widespread acceptance and clinical usage, but it was soon recognized that of themselves the aldosterone antagonists were relatively ineffective. In combination with chlorothiazide drugs and other diuretics, their effectiveness was synergistic and yielded better results than could be anticipated from the summation of actions of the individual drugs.

Further improvement in medical management occurred when ethacrynic acid and furosamide were both found to be significantly more effective than all previously known diuretic agents. Of the two, ethacrynic acid appeared to be the more potent, but furosamide exhibited an unusually broad dose response curve, and in large doses its potency approached that of ethacrynic acid. The physiologic changes induced by these two agents were quite similar; they pointed to a dual site of action in the ascending limb of Henle's loop in the kidney where medullary hypertonicity is normally accomplished and to a second site of action in the distal tubule where urinary dilution is accomplished. These observations indicated a probable qualitative difference between the newer agents and the thiazide diuretics although the overall effects were certainly more similar to the conventional thiazides than to any other type of diuretic agent. If used with appropriate precautions, ethacrynic acid and furosamide promise to be extremely valuable diuretic agents, but the margin of safety is less than one finds with the thiazide drugs. A patient receiving either of these agents must be very carefully observed in order to prevent disastrous and rapid shifts in fluid and electrolyte balance and the development of encephalopathy and coma. Mercurial diuretics may be used cautiously in association with the above agents but only when adequate renal perfusion and urinary output have been established.

The role of depressed intravascular osmotic pressure, so commonly found with cirrhosis, has been emphasized in the pathogenesis of ascites. Therefore, the use of salt-free human serum albumin is extremely important in the depleted patient and should be administered cautiously to restore the serum albumin level to near normal; emphasis should be made, however, of the fact that injudicious use of human serum albumin may cause rapid rises in portal pressure and frequently precipitate bleeding from esophageal varices.

The malnutrition associated with cirrhotic ascites is usually impressive, and the patient appears as a thin, wasted, almost cachectic individual with a huge, tense abdomen and clearly in negative nitrogen balance with a loss of lean body mass. A high carbohydrate intake is imperative even if forced feeding through a soft Penrose tubing is necessary. A high protein intake is important from the nutritional standpoint, but, since portal-systemic shunting is so commonly found with cirrhotic ascites, the induction of encephalopathy is an ever present threat, and protein intake should be increased cautiously by small increments and reduced immediately if asterixis or neurologic symptoms appear.

The type of medical regimen outlined above has been extremely satisfactory in inducing diuresis in most patients with cirrhotic ascites unless they are in the terminal phases of the disease or the hemodynamic component in the pathogenesis is a disproportionate factor. In this latter case or in patients in whom bleeding from esophageal varices does not permit a leisurely medical program, surgical intervention may be required and will be discussed below.

surgical

In order to clarify the selected group of individuals with whom we are dealing when we discuss surgical procedures for cirrhotic ascites, it should be understood that reference is made to two major classes of patients. First are those who are truly intractable to medical therapy but generally not in severe and progressive hepatic decompensation. The second comprises those individuals in whom the onset of severe gastrointestinal bleeding requires immediate consideration for surgical intervention. This latter group, therefore, is one in which the existence of ascites presents an added complication to the primary problem of hemorrhage. The definition of intractability is a point that also requires clarification since this will obviously vary widely with each physician responsible for the management of a patient with ascites. As a generalization, it is not unreasonable to say that ascites might be considered intractable if it is not diminished or dissipated after three to four months of vigorous and consistent medical therapy designed along the guidelines referred to in the preceding section. It has often been said that a year is required in order to evaluate the success or failure of a medical program, but in many instances progressive inanition and complications of diuretic therapy will be lethal. Even in the group of patients who survive, a significant percentage will be completely incapacitated during the entire period.

With these very rough guidelines in mind, one might then proceed to consider what role the surgeon has to play in the management of the patient with severe or intractable cirrhotic ascites. The long history of surgical efforts to dissipate ascites is summarized in Table 5-2. Many ingenious and sometimes bizarre procedures and devices have been employed, but the rather signal lack of success in most instances has made these procedures of historic interest rather than of current significance. Nonetheless, there are occasions when one or another of these procedures or devices might be utilized, and special circumstances for miscellaneous procedures will be referred to again at the end of this section.

Perhaps the most important surgical advance in the treatment of cirrhotic ascites occurred with the revival of shunt surgery in the treatment of this particular complication of cirrhosis. It is of interest to note that the first successful experimental shunt performed by Eck in 1877 was carried out with the concept that it might be applicable to the problem of ascites in man. With the introduction of shunting procedures into clinical usage some 60 years later by Whipple,

TABLE 5-2. Procedures for Ascites

I. Establish collateral
   A. Talma-Morison omentopexy
   B. Spleen in abdominal wall, testicle in peritoneal cavity, excision of parietal peritoneum
II. Reduce portal flow
   A. Arterial ligation
   B. Splenectomy
III. Promote drainage or absorption
   A. Anastomosis of renal pelvis or bladder to peritoneum
   B. Button in subcutaneous tissue
   C. Saphenous vein to peritoneum
   D. "Rectus wick" (divided rectus to peritoneal cavity)
   E. Ileal entectropy
   F. Splenohepatic sinus (Ravdin)
   G. Splenic transposition
IV. Shunt surgery
V. Venous infusion of ascitic fluid
VI. Peritoneal-atrial shunt

Blakemore and Linton, it was hoped that variants of the shunt procedure might prove to be effective in this particular situation. Initially the high mortality in this group of patients and the lack of effectiveness of the end-to-side portacaval shunt in dissipating ascites led to the generally accepted concept that the existence of an appreciable amount of ascites was an actual contraindication to a shunting procedure. With the evolution and understanding of the pathophysiology associated with cirrhotic ascites, however, there was a revival of interest in shunt procedures specifically directed towards alleviation of this problem. Welch and his associates and our group both approached this problem with the concept that one of the major factors in intractable ascites was the existence of an intrahepatic outflow block producing what might be described as a physiologic analogue to the experimental methods of obstructing hepatic outflow and the disease process of bush-tea poisoning in which the hepatic venous outflow is obstructed within the liver itself. Each group reported a series of cases successfully treated by either side-to-side or double shunt, both procedures effecting a combined decompression of the intrahepatic as well as the splanchnic vascular bed. When decompression of the intrahepatic vascular bed is accomplished by any shunting procedure that permits a reversed outflow from the liver to the systemic circulation, an impressive metabolic change occurs with the disappearance of the hyperaldosteronism, a rapidly decreasing excretion of sodium in the urine, a fall in the excretion of potassium and a rapid loss of weight by the dissipation of the ascites. Equally impressive is the rapid restoration of nutritional balance similar to that which is achieved after successful medical therapy. The various types of shunts that have been employed clinically have been diagramed and described elsewhere; it is obvious that every one of these procedures *except* the end-to-side portacaval shunt provides, to varying degrees, an egress route from the intrahepatic vascular and sinusoidal bed, congested by an outflow block, to the low pressure systemic circulation. In retrospect, it is clear why the end-to-side portacaval shunt, which was so commonly employed in the early era of shunt surgery, resulted in extremely unsatisfactory results in patients with ascites; in fact, it was often associated with the development of ascites where none had been present prior to operation.

It should be emphasized strongly, however, that the clinical success and low mortality of combined portal and hepatic decompression in the treatment of cirrhotic ascites depend on careful selection of patients. In those with reasonably good liver function, one might anticipate that hemodynamic factors and an outflow block are prominent in the pathogenesis of the persistent ascites and that it is not purely a manifestation of progressive hepatocellular failure with inability to synthesize albumin and to maintain an adequate intravascular osmotic pressure. With this type of selection and intelligent postoperative management, the results should be good. In Figures 5-2, 5-3 and 5-4 are shown the diagrammatic and photographic representations of the double end-to-side shunt, the dramatic clinical

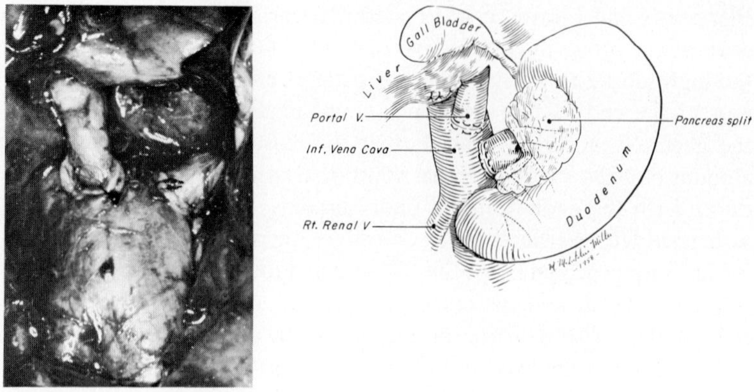

FIG. 5-2. Photographic and diagrammatic representation of the double portacaval shunt used in patients with severe ascites. (Reproduced from McDermott, W. V., Jr.: The Double Portacaval Shunt in the Treatment of Cirrhotic Ascites. Surg. Gynec. Obstet. *110:*457–469, 1960, with permission of the Publishers)

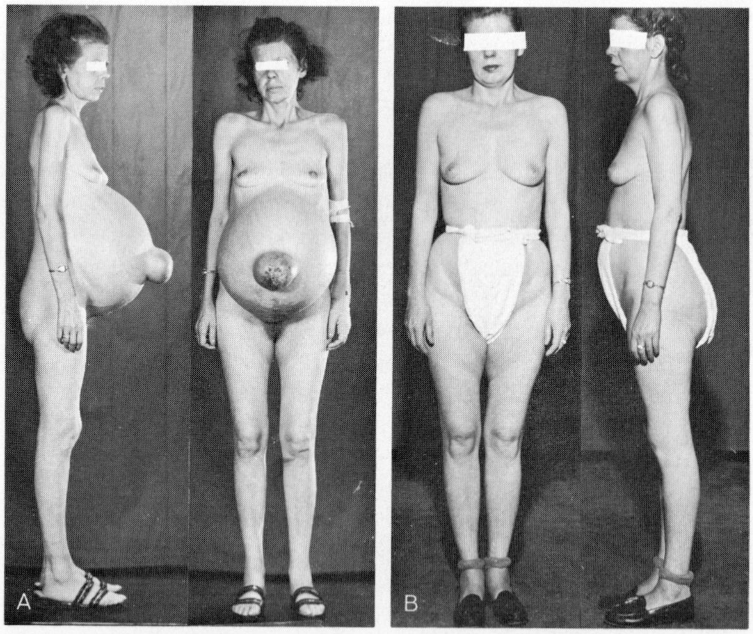

FIG. 5-3. A, Patient with intractable ascites prior to construction of a double portacaval shunt. (Reproduced from McDermott, W. V., Jr.: The Double Portacaval Shunt in the Treatment of Cirrhotic Ascites. Surg. Gynecol. Obstet. *110:*457–469, 1960, with permission of the Publishers). B, Patient four months after surgery; note the absence of ascites and the impressive improvement in nutritional status. (Reproduced from McDermott, W. V., Jr.: The Double Portacaval Shunt in the Treatment of Cirrhotic Ascites. Surg. Gynec. Obstet. *110:*457–469, 1960, with permission of the Publishers)

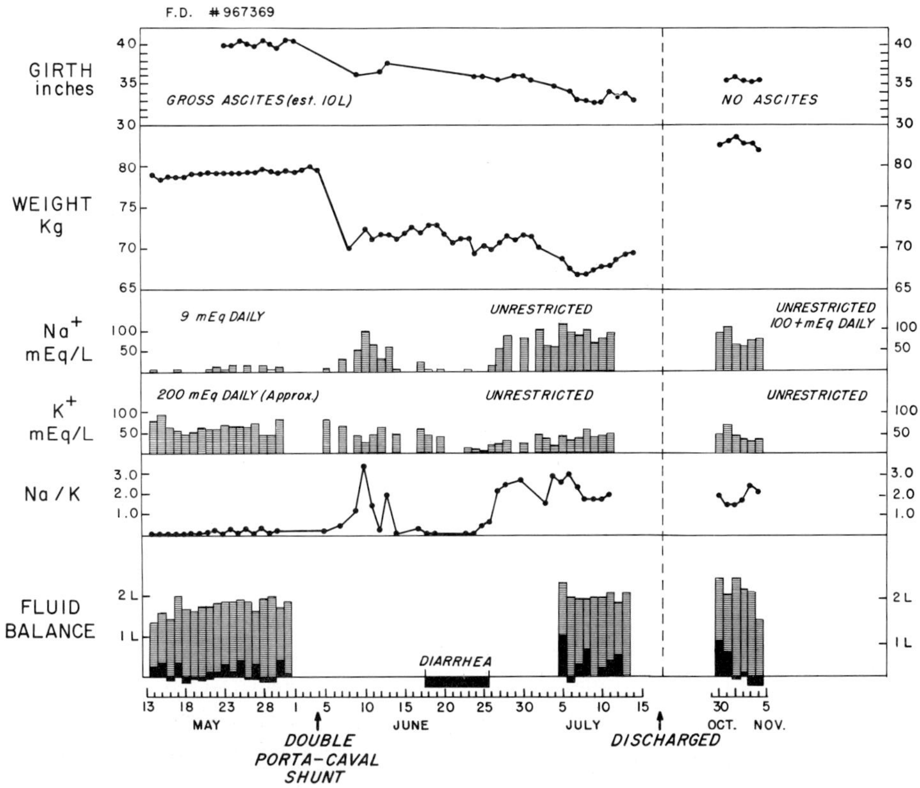

FIG. 5-4. Metabolic chart of patient shown in Figs. 5-3A and 5-3B. (Reproduced from McDermott, W. V., Jr.: The Double Portacaval Shunt in the Treatment of Cirrhotic Ascites. Surg. Gynec. Obstet. *110*:457–469, 1960, with permission of the Publishers)

changes that occur within a few weeks following surgery and the rapid reversal of the abnormal metabolic problems in sodium, potassium and fluid balance.

Several years ago we reviewed 40 patients with intractable ascites in whom various types of shunts had been performed (Table 5-3). Although not a prospective or randomized study, the clinical effectiveness in dissipating ascites of shunts (double or side-to-side portacaval) that provide decompression of the intrahepatic as well as the splanchnic vascular bed is obvious. The splenorenal, which is hemodynamically a smaller side-to-side shunt, is less effective and the end-to-side shunt, which blocks any possible reversal of flow, is least desirable; in fact, construction of an end-to-side portacaval shunt has on several occasions resulted in the development of ascites where it had not existed prior to operation.

Postoperative management is obviously of extreme importance. When the ascites is dissipated during the laparotomy for the construction of a combined decompressing shunt, the immediate postoperative period will be associated with rapid reaccumulation of at least some of the intraperitoneal fluid; why the abnormal pathophysiology is not immediately reversed is not entirely clear, but it may be because the dissection required to construct the shunt leaves a large number of open lymphatics. During this initial period of rapid although variable reaccumulation, the urine output and the specific gravity should be followed at two-hour intervals and maintained at an adequate volume and a moderate degree of concentration. This may require many units of plasma or salt-free albumin during the first 24 hours, but eventually stabilization occurs as indicated by the maintenance of an adequate urine output and the cessation of rapid weight gain. If adequate volume replacement is not carried out, one encounters the typical azotemia and, ultimately, death. It should be emphasized, however, that the renal problem in this instance is quite different from that seen with fulminant hepatic failure and is identical to that encountered with inadequately treated burns. After stabilization one can anticipate the increasing appearance of sodium in the urine and progressive dissipation of the reaccumulated ascites; this is usually complete within three weeks, and the patient may leave the hospital without salt restriction or the necessity for any diuretic program.

Before concluding, it should be pointed out that there are instances in which procedures other than shunting may be employed for ascites. For example, in a patient in whom intractable ascites develops after an end-to-side portacaval shunt, there is no way of decompressing the congested intrahepatic bed except by scarification of the surface of the liver with the hope of developing collaterals to the diaphragm or by the construction of an isolated ileal segment, a procedure referred to by Neuman and Hinton as ileal entectropy. In the congenital Chiari syndrome, construction of an adequate shunt in an infant or very young child is not feasible, and transposition of the spleen into the chest with successful dissipation of the ascites has been reported. In patients whose poor liver function precludes any type of operative procedure, the constant reinfusion of collected ascitic fluid in association with the administration of ethacrynic acid or one of the other

TABLE 5-3. Results of Shunt Surgery in 40 Patients with Intractable Ascites

	Number of Cases	Hospital Deaths	Survivors	Successful (No Further Ascites) Number of Cases	Successful (No Further Ascites) % of Original Group
Double or side-to-side portacaval	17	2 (12%)	15	14	82%
End-to-side portacaval	8	2 (25%)	6	2	25%
Splenorenal	15	5 (33%)	10	7	47%

diuretics may turn the corner for the patient just as the insertion of the device for a peritoneal-atrial shunt as described by Eiseman may do on a more long term basis.

bibliography

Atkinson, M.: Ascites in liver disease. Postgrad. Med. J., *32:*482-485, 1956.

Atkinson, M., and Losowsky, M. S.: The mechanism of ascites formation in chronic liver disease. Quart. J. Med., *N.S.30:*153-166, 1961.

Baggenstoss, A. H., and Cain, J. C.: The hepatic hilar lymphatics of man. Their relation to ascites. New Eng. J. Med., *256:*531-535, 1957.

Bartter, F. C., Biglieri, E. G., Pronove, P., and Delea, C. S.: Effect of changes in intravascular volume on aldosterone secretion in man. *In* Muller, A. F. and O'Connor, C. M. (Eds.): An International Symposium on Aldosterone. Boston, Little Brown and Company, 1958, pp. 100-110.

Berman, J. K., Koenig, H., and Muller, L. P.: Ligation of hepatic and splenic arteries in treatment of portal hypertension. Ligation in atrophic cirrhosis of the liver. Arch. Surg., *63:*379-389, 1951.

Bras, G., and Hill, K. R.: Veno-occlusive disease of the liver. Essential pathology. Lancet, *2:*161-163, 1956.

Bras, G., Berry, D. M., and György, P.: Plants as aetiological factor in veno-occlusive disease of the liver. Lancet, *1:*960-962, 1957.

Britton, R. C.: The hepatic outflow tract and ascites: Angiographic and cinefluorographic studies. Amer. J. Gastroent., *44:*443-454, 1965.

Britton, R. C., Brown, C. H., and Shirey, E. K.: Intrahepatic veno-occlusive disease in cirrhosis with chronic ascites. Diagnosis by hepatic phlebography and results of surgical treatment. Ann. Surg., *158:*370-382, 1963.

Cameron, J. L., Anderson, R. P., and Zuidema, G. D: Pancreatic ascites. Surg. Gynec. Obstet., *125:*328-332, 1967.

Cameron, J. L., Brawley, R. K., Bender, H. W., and Zuidema, G. D.: The treatment of pancreatic ascites. Ann. Surg., *170:*668-676, 1969.

Davidson, C. S.: Cirrhosis of the liver treated with prolonged sodium restrictions. Improvement in nutrition, hepatic function, and portal hypertension. J. A. M. A., *159:*1257-1261, 1955.

Drapanas, T., Schenk, W. G., Jr., Pollack, E. L., and Stewart, J. D.: Hepatic hemodynamics in experimental ascites. Ann. Surg., *152:*705-716, 1960.

Dumont, A. E., and Mulholland, J. H.: Flow rate and composition of thoracic-duct lymph in patients with cirrhosis. New Eng. J. Med., *263:*471-474, 1960.

Dumont, A. E., and Mulholland, J. H.: Alterations in thoracic duct lymph flow in hepatic cirrhosis: significance in portal hypertension. Ann. Surg., *156:*668-677, 1962.

Eisenmenger, W. J., Blondheim, S. H., Bongiovanni, A. M., and Kunkel, H. G.: Electrolyte studies on patients with cirrhosis of the liver. J. Clin. Invest., *29:*1491-1499, 1950.

Giuseffi, J., et al.: Effect of bilateral adrenalectomy in a patient with massive ascites and postnecrotic cirrhosis. New Eng. J. Med., *257:*796-803, 1957.

Hyatt, R. E., and Smith, J. R.: The mechanism of ascites. A physiologic appraisal. Amer. J. Med., *16:*434-448, 1954.

Jefferson, N. C., and Necheles, H.: Evolution of vascular ligations in reversing experimental ascites. Amer. J. Surg., *85:*529-533, 1953.

Laragh, J. H., Cannon, P. J., Stason, W. B., and Heinemann, H. O.: Physiologic and clinical observations on furosemide and ethacrynic acid. Ann. N.Y. Acad. Sci., *139:*453-465, 1966.

Losowsky, M. S., and Atkinson, M.: Intravenous albumin in the treatment of diuretic-resistant ascites in portal cirrhosis. Lancet, *2:*386-389, 1961.

Losowsky, M. S., and Davidson, C. S.: The source of ascitic fluid in cirrhosis of the liver. Arch. Int. Med., *110:*279-282, 1962.

Losowsky, M. S., Jones, D. P., Lieber, C. S., and Davidson, C. S.: Local factors in ascites formation during sodium retention in cirrhosis. New Eng. J. Med., *268:*651-653, 1963.

Madden, J. L., Loré, J. M., Jr., Gerold, F. P., and David, J. M.: The pathogenesis of ascites and a consideration of its treatment. Surg. Gynec. Obstet., *99:*385-391, 1954.

Mallet-Guy, P., Devic, G., Feroldi, J., et Desjacques, P.: Étude expérimentale des ascites. Sténoses veineuses post-hépatiques et transposition du foie dans le thorax. Lyon Chir., *49:*153-172, 1954.

McDermott, W. V., Jr.: The treatment of cirrhotic ascites by combined hepatic and portal decompression. New Eng. J. Med., *259:*897-901, 1958.

McDermott, W. V., Jr., and Brown, H.: Ascites. *In* Degraff, A. C., and Creger, W. P. (Eds.): Annual Review of Medicine. Palo Alto, Calif., Annual Reviews, Inc., 1964, vol. 15, pp. 79-92.

McKee, F. W., Schilling, J. A., Tishkoff, G. H., and Hyatt, R. E.: Experimental ascites. Effects of sodium chloride and protein intake on protein metabolism of dogs with constricted inferior vena cava. Surg. Gynec. Obstet., *89:*529-540, 1949.

Moore, R. M., Singleton, A. O., Jr., and Pickett, W. H.: Splenic artery ligation in palliation of ascites. Ann. Surg., *131:*774-780, 1950.

Nebesar, R. A., Kornblith, P. L., Pollard, J. J., and Michels, N. A.: Celiac and Superior Mesenteric Arteries. A Correlation of Angiograms and Dissections. Boston, Little Brown and Company, 1969, 226 pp.

Neumann, C. G., Adie, G. C., and Hinton, J. W.: The absorption of ascitic fluid by means of ileo-entectropy in patients with advanced cirrhosis. Ann. Surg., *146:*700-705, 1957.

Neumann, C. G., Braunwald, N. S., and Hinton, J. W.: The absorption of ascitic fluid by a pedicled flap of intestinal mucosa exposed within the peritoneal cavity. Plast. Reconstr. Surg., *17:*189-195, 1956.

Orloff, M. J., and Snyder, G. B.: Experimental ascites. I. Production of ascites by gradual occlusion of the hepatic veins with an internal vena cava cannula. Surgery, *50:*789-797, 1961.

Orloff, M. J., et al.: Hepatic regulation of aldosterone secretion by a humoral mediator. Surgery, *58:*225-247, 1965.

Reemtsma, K., Carlson, R. E., Habif, D. V., and Barker, H. G.: Changes in sodium metabolism following portacaval shunts in patients with cirrhosis and ascites. Surg. Forum, *7:*422-425, 1957.

Rienhoff, W. F., Jr.: Ligation of the hepatic and splenic arteries in the treatment of portal hypertension with a report of six cases. Preliminary report. Bull. Johns Hopkins Hosp., *88:*368-375, 1951.

Rosato, E. F., Berkowitz, H. D., and Roberts, B.: Bile ascites. Surg. Gynec. Obstet., *130:*494-496, 1970.

Schaffner, F., et al.: Budd-Chiari syndrome caused by a web in the inferior vena cava. Amer. J. Med., *42:*838-843, 1967.

Schinaberger, J. H., and Galambos, J. T.: Management of "refractory" ascites. Based on correction of specific physiologic lesions. Amer. J. Gastroent., *41:*499-518, 1964.

Schreiner, G. E., and Bloomer, H. A.: Effect of chlorothiazide on the edema of cirrhosis, nephrosis, congestive heart failure and chronic renal insufficiency. New Eng. J. Med., *257:*1016-1022, 1957.

Schwartz, S. I., and Adesola, A. O.: Influence of vasoactive agents on ascites. Surgery, *58:*215-224, 1965.

Seldin, D. W.: Introductory remarks. *In* The physiology of diuretic agents. Ann. N.Y. Acad. Sci., *139:*275, 1966.

Shear, L., Ching, S., and Gabuzda, G. J.: Compartmentalization of ascites and edema in patients with hepatic cirrhosis. New Eng. J. Med., *282:* 1391-1396, 1970.

Sherlock, S., Walker, J. G., Senewiratne, B., and Scott, A.: The complications of diuretic therapy in patients with cirrhosis. Ann. N.Y. Acad. Sci., *139:*497-505, 1966.

Symposium on Liver Disease: II. Treatment of ascites and hepatic insufficiency. Amer. J. Gastroent., *38:*15-39, 1962.

Teague, F. B., Jr., Warren, W. D., and Respess, J. C.: Vascular physiology in portal hypertension with ascites. Clinical and experimental studies and role of portocaval shunt. Ann. Surg., *163:*112-120, 1966.

Theron, P., and Allan, J. C.: Ascites: A clinical and experimental study. Acta Med. Scand., *152* (Suppl. 306):145-154, 1955.

Volwiler, W., Bollman, J. L., and Grindlay, J. H.: A comparison of two types of experimental ascites. Proc. Staff Meet. Mayo Clin., *25:*31-33, 1950.

Volwiler, W., Grindlay, J. H., and Bollman, J. L.: The relation of portal vein pressure to the formation of ascites—an experimental study. Gastroenterology, *14:*40-55, 1950.

Walker, W. G.: Indications and contraindications for diuretic therapy. Ann. N.Y. Acad. Sci., *139:*481-496, 1966.

Wantz, G. E.: Ascites in liver disease. Pathogenesis and treatment. Surg. Clin. N. Amer., *38:*407-420, 1958.

Welch, C. S., Attarian, E., and Welch, H. F.: The treatment of ascites by side to side portacaval shunt. Bull. N.Y. Acad. Med., *34:*249-255, 1958.

Whittlesey, R. H., Ingram, P. R., and Riker, W. L.: Chylous ascites in childhood. Report of five cases. Ann. Surg., *142:*1013-1020, 1955.

Witte, C. L., et al.: Dual origin of ascites in hepatic cirrhosis. Surg. Gynec. Obstet., *129:*1027-1033, 1969.

Wolfman, E. F., Jr., Zuidema, G. D., and Child, C. G., III: Urinary sodium and aldosterone excretion following portocaval shunts for cirrhosis of liver and portal hypertension: Effect of end-to-side and side-to-side anastomoses in 16 cases. Ann. Surg., *164:*538-546, 1966.

Zeppa, R., and Womack, N. A.: Humoral control of hepatic lymph flow. Surgery, *54:*37-44, 1963.

Diagnosis and Management of Bleeding Esophageal Varices

CHAPTER 6

The occurrence of bleeding from varices in the esophagus is a common and serious complication of portal hypertension. While bleeding from this source is common in extrahepatic portal bed block and in the type of presinusoidal intrahepatic block seen with schistosomiasis, the most frequent cause of this problem in the continental United States is the existence of one of the types of portal cirrhosis. Therefore, in this particular discussion, attention will be focused on the patient with established intrahepatic disease who bleeds from esophageal varices. Many of the principles of diagnosis and treatment in this group are equally applicable to other causes of portal hypertension, but since the presence of cirrhosis presents added problems, adjustments in treatment towards less complicated problems can be made easily.

In the presence of cirrhosis, this type of bleeding is frequently catastrophic and, as a matter of fact, is often merely the terminal event in progressive hepatic decompensation. The combination of massive blood loss, hypovolemia and the multiple metabolic disorders associated with the presence of liver disease makes this particular clinical problem an unusually challenging and difficult one. Treatment must be focused on both control of the exsanguinating hemorrhage and correction of the metabolic disorders, of which the most common is the encephalopathy already discussed, associated with portal-systemic shunting and hyperammoniemia.

diagnosis of bleeding esophageal varices

The existence of esophageal varices as a source of upper gastrointestinal bleeding must be suspected in any patient with a history of alcoholism or with the stigmata of liver disease (liver palms, spider angiomata, hepatosplenomegaly, abdominal wall collateral circulation, ascites, gynecomastia and testicular atrophy). The exact diagnosis is particularly difficult, however, because many patients with chronic alcoholism bleed from gastritis; also, duodenal ulcer is found in approximately 10 per cent of patients with cirrhosis of the liver. In addition, portal hypertension may develop in the presence of an intrahepatic portal bed block that is characterized primarily by periportal fibrosis rather than destruction or disruption of hepatic parenchyma; in these instances the stigmata of liver disease may be absent, liver function tests remarkably normal and no overt physical or biochemical abnormalities present to suggest the possibility of portal hypertension.

history and physical examination

An accurate history and a careful physical examination will provide many of the keys to the establishment of an exact diagnosis. The nutritional and social history of the patient, presence or absence of gastrointestinal symptoms and presence or absence of the stigmata of liver disease are all of great importance. Particular reference, however, should be made to obtaining an exact history of the *nature of the bleeding.* Very commonly there is no true hematemesis associated with bleeding esophageal varices, and the patient will give a story of bright red blood suddenly welling out of his mouth rather than an actual bout of emesis with blood in the gastric contents.

LABORATORY STUDIES. A *Bromsulphalein test* should be done immediately; this is an extremely sensitive test of hepatocellular function. A normal reading will exclude the presence of liver disease, but increased retention may be only a reflection of decreased hepatic blood flow; we have seen quite significant abnormalities in this particularly sensitive test in patients who have no intrinsic liver disease. *Other liver function tests* should be obtained, particularly as a base line, but many of them will not be available as emergency procedures. Protein characterization is important, and decreased albumin and increased globulin levels are particularly characteristic of cirrhosis. *Blood ammonia level* is especially valuable under these circumstances if it can be obtained as an emergency procedure as either a quantitative or qualitative determination. In contradistinction to the BSP test, the level of blood ammonia is a very unsatisfactory index of liver function because of the extreme degree of reserve in the mechanism of urea synthesis. Rather, hyperammoniemia in the peripheral blood is a very sensitive index of the degree of portal-systemic shunting, and, therefore, if one sees a patient with well compensated liver disease and hyperammoniemia subsequent to gastrointestinal bleeding, there is almost *prima facie* evidence that extensive portal-systemic shunting exists and esophageal varices are present. Therefore, one has two relatively simple tests, one of which functions as a very sensitive index of hepatocellular function and the other as an index of portal-systemic shunting. Evaluated together, they are particularly valuable.

In Figure 6-1, the results of a study of changes in Bromsulphalein retention and peripheral blood ammonia concentrations in patients with massive upper gastrointestinal bleeding are shown diagrammatically. In patients who proved to be bleeding from esophageal varices, all the ammonia levels were elevated except for one individual who was under treatment with a broad spectrum antibiotic. The BSP levels were invariably higher than normal in patients with liver disease but were not infrequently high in those without either liver disease or esophageal varices.

Coagulation studies should be obtained immediately as in any case of hemorrhage; a prothrombin deficiency ordinarily exists that may or may not be correctable by the intravenous administration of vitamin K. Many other coagulation defects occur with cirrhosis of the liver and can be evaluated individually. From the practical point of view, however, the major therapeutic approach involves the administration of fresh blood rather than units that have been stored for days or weeks in the blood bank. Thrombocytopenia is commonly seen attendant upon the hypersplenism of portal hypertension. This is of clinical importance only if the platelets fall below 50,000 per cu. mm., but if the smear or platelet count indicates a significant deficiency, this is correctable by utilizing fresh blood with adequate platelets in

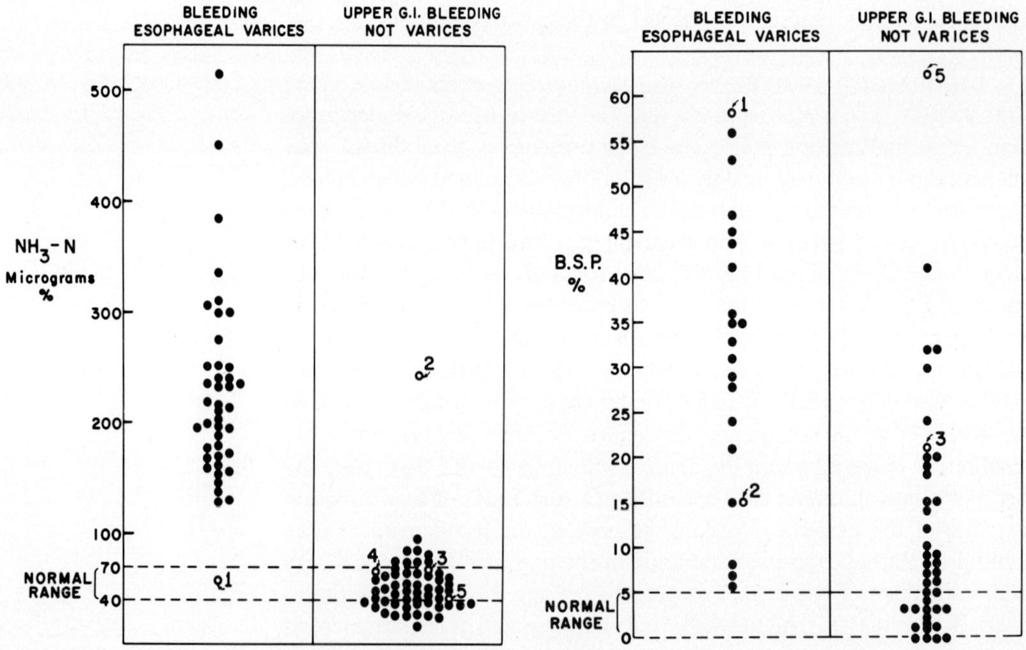

FIG. 6-1. Comparison of blood ammonia levels and BSP retention in a series of patients with upper gastrointestinal hemorrhage. (Reproduced from McDermott, W. V., Jr.: A Simple Discriminatory Test for Upper Gastrointestinal Hemorrhage. N. Eng. J. Med. *257*:1161–1164, 1957, with permission of the Publishers)

terms of number and function or giving actual platelet transfusions. *Fibrinolysins* occur with liver disease and particularly with the various complications, of which bleeding esophageal varices are the ones under consideration. Significant fibrinolysis can be detected in a very simple way early after the patient's admission and, if present, epsilon-aminocaproic acid should be given in an attempt to control this particular aspect of the coagulation abnormality.

Splenic pulp manometry has been utilized and recommended by Rousselot in the diagnosis of bleeding varices. This procedure can be carried out quite simply on an emergency floor, and in the series reported by Rousselot, a pressure level of 300 mm. of water was the dividing line between those patients who proved to be bleeding from the esophageal veins and those who were not. This recommendation is supported by our own observations in elective cases in which it was found extremely unusual for any patient with portal hypertension to have bled from varices until the pressure reached approximately this level or higher. Therefore, if one finds a relatively low splenic pulp pressure, the diagnosis of bleeding esophageal varices can be excluded unless the patient is in severe shock and even if small varices are detectable by other diagnostic means. If one has the facilities available at the time of the manometry, this can be followed by a splenoportography (Fig. 6-2), which may give added diagnostic infor-

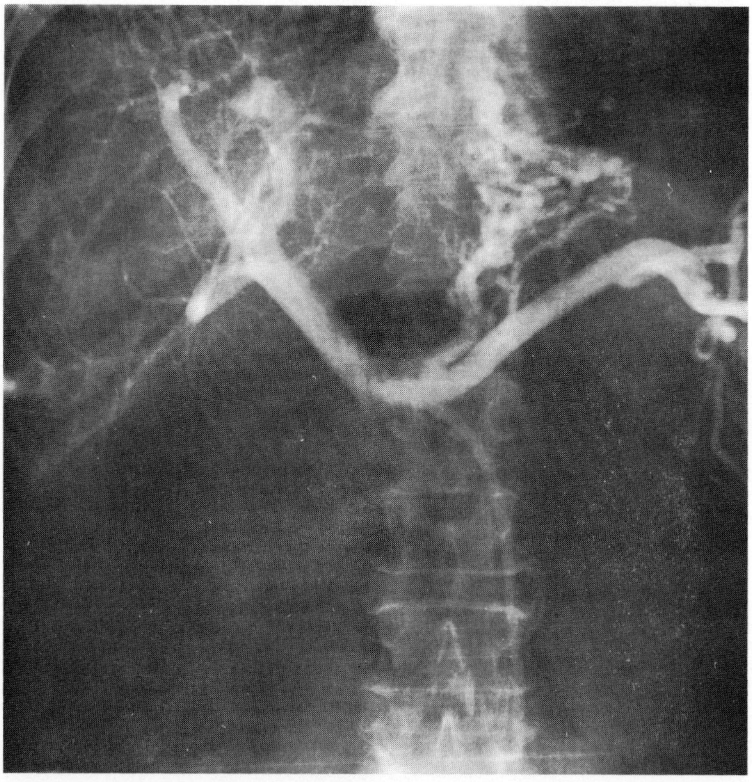

FIG. 6-2. Splenoportogram demonstrating esophageal varices

mation relative to the presence or absence of esophageal varices and the patency of the portal vein.

endoscopy

The use of esophagoscopy and gastroscopy is of great value in any case of upper gastrointestinal bleeding, but its usefulness is directly related to the skill and experience of the operator. It is also unsuccessful in patients with massive bleeding since the view of the observer may be obscured to a degree that renders the procedure fruitless.

radiographic techniques

Reference has already been made to *splenoportography,* and the more recent introduction of *selective arteriography* has been an extremely valuable adjunct to diagnosis and may prove to be useful in treatment. A catheter inserted into the celiac axis followed by the introduction of a solution of 50 per cent Hypaque will give excellent visualization of the arterial supply to the liver, spleen and upper splanchnic area. In the delayed phase, one can usually obtain good visualization of the splenic and portal veins, and esophageal varices may be demonstrated at that time. The pooling in the gastrointestinal tract of radiopaque material will frequently provide direct and exact information as to the location of the point of bleeding. Once diagnostic studies have been completed, the catheter may be left in position for regular infusions of surgical Pituitrin. Perhaps the most commonly used diagnostic tool is the *upper gastrointestinal series.* If the patient is not in severe shock or comatose, and if time permits, this procedure has a high degree of accuracy in determining the presence or absence of esophageal varices and also in demonstrating and locating other lesions of the upper gastrointestinal tract.

Balloon tamponade, a method that is still the most widely used in the control of bleeding from esophageal varices, can also function diagnostically. If by any combination of the various diagnostic techniques described above, the location of the source of the massive gastrointestinal bleeding is still uncertain, the introduction of the double balloon tube may be extremely useful in determining at least the organic location of the bleeding site. Although tamponade is usually thought of in terms of compressing and controlling esophageal varices, it may also be effective in the Mallory-Weiss syndrome and other types of esophageal disorders or in high-lying gastric ulcers. Therefore, the abrupt cessation of the gastrointestinal hemorrhage upon inflation of the balloons should be considered as suggesting but not conclusively demonstrating that the varices were, in fact, the source of the hemorrhage.

the treatment of bleeding esophageal varices

control of hemorrhage

Clearly the key to management of the entire problem is control of hemorrhage, although the details of methods of correction of the numerous metabolic abnormalities are clearly a vital part of the overall problem. Not infrequently hemorrhage from esophageal varices will stop spontaneously as the portal pressure drops with hypovolemia. It is important to maintain organ perfusion at a reasonable oxygen-carrying capacity, but it is also important not to overtransfuse the patient. In fact, a moderate degree of hypovolemia will probably contribute to spontaneous cessation of bleeding. In general, we prefer to keep the hematocrit between 25 and 30% and to sustain adequate organ perfusion by monitoring the urine output and maintaining it at a level of at least 20 cc. per hour. If the bleeding ceases spontaneously, the patient then moves into the category for consideration of a later elective portal-systemic shunt.

If, however, the bleeding is exsanguinating or continuing, active measures must be instituted. *Vasopressin* or *surgical Pituitrin,* given intravenously or through a catheter left in the superior mesenteric artery after diagnostic arteriography (celiac), serves as a pharmacologic method of lowering the portal pressure by diminishing splanchnic inflow; if it is given rapidly in dosages of 20 U. in 200 cc. of fluid, the pharmacologic effect will last only 20 to 30 minutes but the infusion may be repeated at frequent intervals. It would appear that the rationale behind this approach is satisfactory, and on occasions clinical results seem to be gratifying. This type of approach is obviously very difficult to evaluate, however. A randomized study by Davidson of the use of surgical Pituitrin in patients with bleeding varices demonstrated that while individual episodes of bleeding were controlled temporarily, there was no increased overall salvage in terms of a patient's ultimately leaving the hospital alive and well.

If this type of pharmacologic approach is not satisfactory or if the bleeding is so massive that further immediate intervention is required, the classic and still most widely applied method of treatment is the use of *balloon tamponade.* A number of different balloon tubes have been designed, but in our opinion the most satisfactory is based on the original Sengstaken-Blakemore tube, which provides for double compression through gastric and esophageal balloons (Fig. 6-3). The details of the use of this balloon tube are extremely important. Clearly, the balloon and tube should be checked carefully before insertion. As the tube is introduced through the nose and ultimately into the stomach, the gastric balloon, which should have a capacity of at least 300 cc., is then inflated and drawn snugly up against the hiatus. The tubing is then fixed in place in the nose without traction with a sponge rubber cuff to prevent erosion of the nasal alae (a number of different types of head gear have been used to hold the balloon in place and,

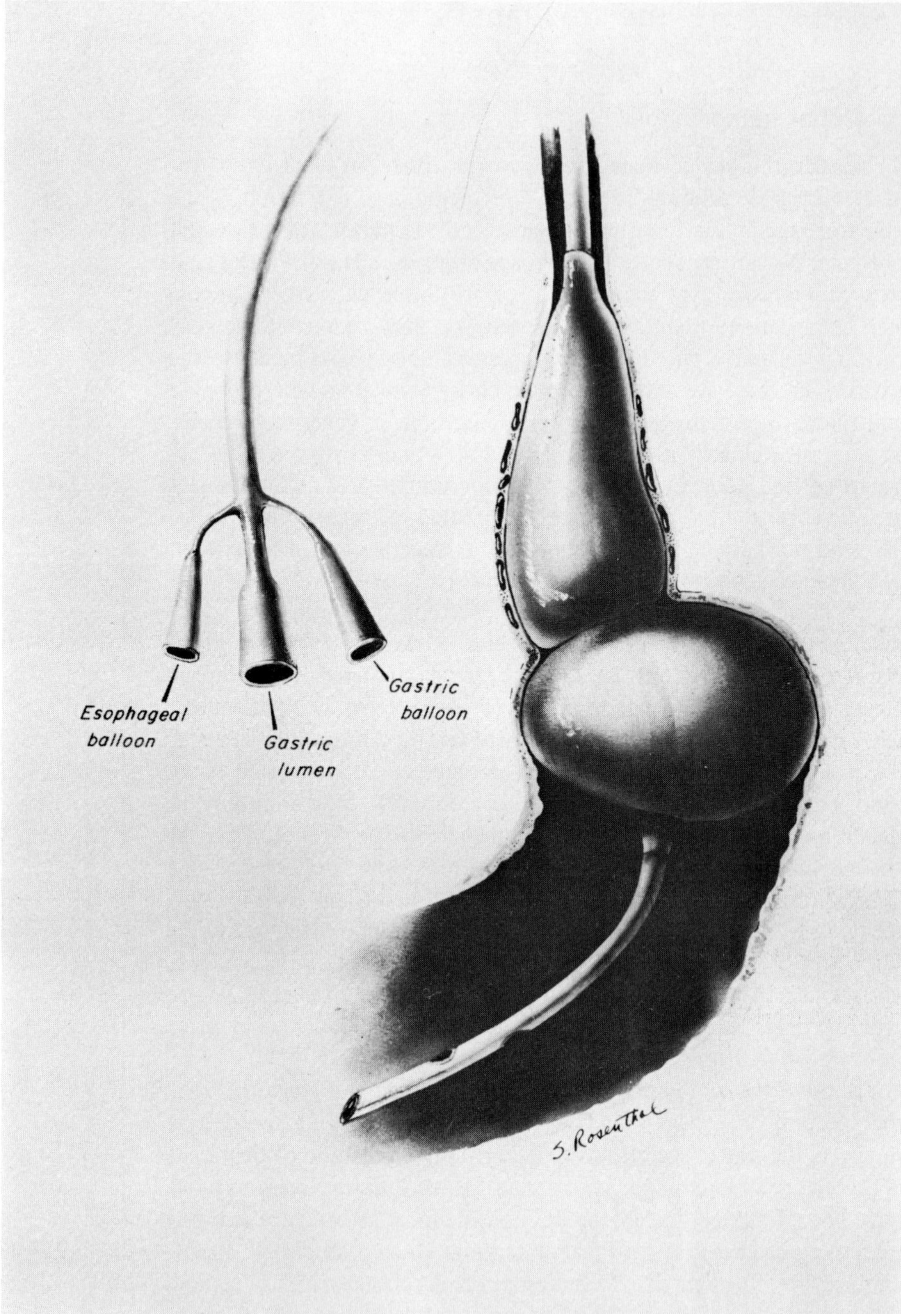

FIG. 6-3. Diagram of the proper placement of the double (Sengstaken-Blakemore) tube

if available, are certainly very satisfactory means of fixation). Following fixation of the gastric balloon, the esophageal balloon can be inflated and the inlet tubing connected via a Y attachment with a manometer and a syringe. The pressure in the esophageal balloon should be maintained at a level between 30 and 40 mm. of mercury. Careful attention to monitoring of this pressure is essential to prevent either loss of pressure with further bleeding, or erosion or rupture of the esophagus because of overinflation. Since the Sengstaken-Blakemore tube has no orifices for suction above the balloons, it is useful to introduce a small suction tubing through the other nasal orifice into the upper esophagus in order to withdraw, by suction, secretions and any minor continued oozing that may occur.

If the diagnosis of bleeding esophageal varices is correct, balloon tamponade carried out in this fashion will ordinarily control the hemorrhage; if it does not, it means that the bleeding is coming from some other source or that the balloon tube is inadequately positioned. Often the balloon can be palpated in the epigastrium, but it is probably wise to check its position by x-ray visualization, particularly if the insertion seems unsatisfactory in any way. If bleeding is controlled by tamponade, one should leave this in position for about 48 hours and then gradually release pressure, first from the esophageal balloon and then finally from the gastric balloon, leaving the tube in place and on 1½ pounds of gastric suction to determine the presence or absence of recurrent bleeding. If no bleeding recurs after a further 24 hours, the balloon can be removed, the patient started on increasing bland feedings and, hopefully, brought to consideration of elective shunt.

If bleeding recurs successively after several attempts to release the balloon pressure on the esophagus or if the balloon tamponade does not control bleeding, one has recourse only to direct *transthoracic ligation of the esophageal varices* or abdominal exploration if the actual diagnosis is still in doubt. Figure 6-4 shows the general approach to transthoracic ligation of varices, and this procedure may often tide over an individual until he can be brought into condition for elective shunt surgery. After adequate ligation of the usual three rows of esophageal varices, hemorrhage is usually controlled for three to six weeks. This will allow a period of restoration of nutrition, which is so often deficient in the alcoholic patient, dissipation of ascites and general improvement in liver function prior to consideration of elective shunt. If abdominal exploration is indicated because of doubt of the original diagnosis, the usual procedures in a laparotomy for upper gastrointestinal bleeding of unknown origin are carried out with gastrotomy and careful search of the gastrointestinal tract for the bleeding site. Varices may be ligated from the abdominal route, but this is technically very difficult because of the overlying inflexible cirrhotic left lobe of the liver that so often interferes with adequate exposure of the gastroesophageal junction. An additional disadvantage to the abdominal approach is the necessity for dissipation of any

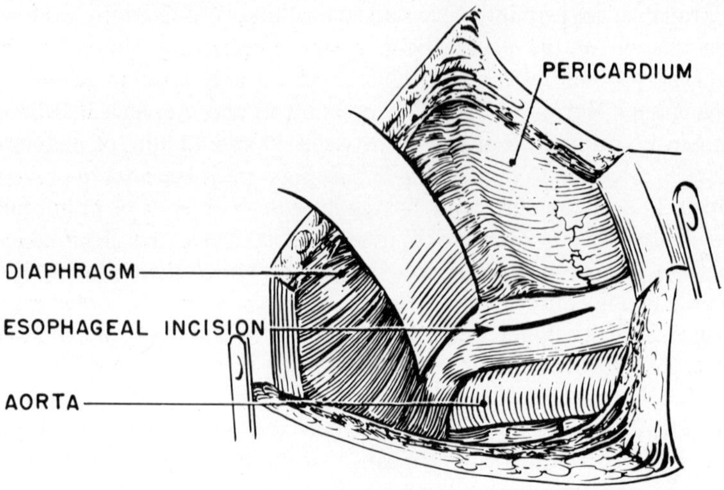

FIG. 6-4. Surgical approach to transthoracic ligation of esophageal varices

accumulated ascites, which will then rapidly reaccumulate during the postoperative period and add to the metabolic problems.

The *urgent shunt* has received considerable attention during the past few years. We have avoided the term "emergency shunt" because a preliminary period of temporary control of bleeding and correction of metabolic abnormalities is almost invariably required before a shunt can be contemplated with any hope of successful outcome. A shunt constructed in the presence of an intestinal tract full of blood provides the perfect pathophysiologic mechanism for hyperammoniemia and hepatic encephalopathy. Therefore, prior to construction of an urgent shunt the bleeding must be controlled by balloon tamponade or other methods, the gut cleansed of blood by cathartics and enemas, intestinal antibiotics initiated, blood volume deficit corrected and adequate renal function restored. Experience over the past few years has led most surgeons to the conclusion that the urgent shunt is applicable only

TABLE 6-1. Clinical and Laboratory Classification of Patients with Cirrhosis in Terms of Hepatic Functional Reserve*

Group Designation	A (minimal)	B (moderate)	C (advanced)
Serum bilirubin† (mg.%)	Below 2.0	2.0–3.0	Over 3.0
Serum albumin (gm.%)	Over 3.5	3.0–3.5	Under 3.0
Ascites	None	Easily controlled	Poorly controlled
Neurologic disorder	None	Minimal	Advanced, "coma"
Nutrition	Excellent	Good	Poor, "wasting"

*From C. G. Child, III: The Hepatic Circulation and Portal Hypertension. Philadelphia, W. B. Saunders Co., 1954.
†Equivocal in biliary cirrhosis.

TABLE 6-2. Method of Calculating Liver Index

Rating for liver index	0	1	2	3	4
Bromsulphalein % retention	<4	<10	<20	<30	<30
Albumin (gm. %)	>3.9	<4.0	<3.5	<3.0	<2.5
Van den Bergh (mg. %)	<1.0	<1.5	<3.0	<6.0	>5.9
Alkaline phosphatase (Bodansky units)	<4.0	<6.0	<15	<30	<29
Cephalin flocculation (48 hours)	0	1	2	3	4
Prothrombin time (% of normal)	>80	<80	<60	<40	<20

to the patients with bleeding esophageal varices who can be placed in the A category as defined by Child (Table 6-1) or with a liver index between 0 and 2 by our classification (Table 6-2). In general, this refers to a patient without jaundice or significant ascites who has a prothrombin time greater than 30 per cent of normal, whose serum albumin level is greater than 3.0 gm. per 100 ml. and who has no significant other disease to complicate the picture.

The overall results in terms of mortality in this catastrophic disease are discouraging. In any series that is completely unselected and includes patients who bleed within the hospital during the terminal phase of liver disease, the mortality rate has been in the range of 60 per cent or higher. In our own randomized study (Table 6-3), which included even terminal patients, the overall mortality was 71 per cent, and there was no significant difference in results between initial treatment with balloon tamponade and Pituitrin alone, transthoracic ligation of varices and urgent shunt. Without going into all the details of this particular study, all patients who were diagnosed by whatever means as bleeding from esophageal varices were admitted to the study. Prior to randomization, they were classified as either good risk or fair to poor. In the operative categories, all patients were not operated upon since clearly one could not consider a decision whether a patient could possibly tolerate surgery that was based purely on random charts. Nevertheless, if a patient who was randomized into one of the operative groups died without surgery, he was classified, for purposes of the study, as an operative death. This avoided any type of selection that might favor surgical approach. Further analysis

TABLE 6-3. Mortality Figures in Which Choice of Treatment Was Determined by Random Selection

Treatment of Choice (by Random)	Balloon Tamponade		Ligation of Varices		Urgent Shunt	
Category of Risk (Child)	A or B	C	A or B	C	A or B	C
Survived	5	1	6	1	5	2
Died	7	7	8	5	9	10
Total	20		18		26	
Died	14		13		19	
Mortality	70%		73%		73%	

of this study would indicate, however, that patients in the A category will do well with an urgent shunt while patients in the C category will rarely if ever tolerate any type of surgery. Decision is frequently difficult in the intermediate group referred to as the B category in which some of the better patients may be considered for urgent shunt and some of the poorer group should not be treated surgically in any way. This leaves a relatively small group of patients in whom transthoracic ligation of varices is probably the treatment of choice as a temporizing measure.

correction of metabolic abnormalities

Of equal importance with the control of hemorrhage from esophageal varices is the correction of metabolic abnormalities that are so intimately associated with this particular problem. Of primary importance is the restoration and maintenance of blood volume in order to avoid the adverse effects of decreased hepatic blood flow and the possibility of acute tubular necrosis secondary to decreased renal perfusion. Ordinarily, the oliguria or anuria seen with bleeding varices is the result of hypovolemia, but the somewhat nebulous hepatorenal syndrome, which will be covered in more detail elsewhere, occasionally complicates the picture if liver function has deteriorated to a serious degree. The patient with bleeding esophageal varices will often have multiple *clotting defects.* The increased *prothrombin time* is characteristically seen in cirrhosis of the liver but does not present a serious clinical deficit unless it falls below 30 per cent of normal. Intravenous vitamin K should be given although if the defect is in the synthetic function in the liver the abnormal prothrombin time may well be unresponsive. *Thrombocytopenia* is commonly associated with portal hypertension when there is severe fibrocongestive splenomegaly and sequestration of circulating blood elements; again, this common defect is not clinically significant unless the platelets by count are below 50,000 per cu. mm. Nonetheless, an initial moderate defect in platelets will rapidly become serious if bleeding continues and the blood replacement is confined to bank blood with defective platelet function. A number of other defects in the clotting mechanism have been described in association with liver disease in this period in this particular clinical problem, and details are of academic interest only because the practical way of correcting these multiple defects, including those in prothrombin synthesis and in platelet deficiency, consists of replacement of blood volume with fresh blood as soon as possible. The presence of *circulating fibrinolysin* can be easily detected by bedside observation of the lysis of a formed clot; by the administration of epsilon-aminocaproic acid, it may be possible to control this process. A consumptive coagulopathy is more likely to be associated with fulminant hepatic failure than with the clinical syndrome of bleeding esophageal varices, but it must be considered, particularly if there is superimposed infection with gram-negative organisms.

Portal-systemic encephalopathy is a very common phenomenon with bleeding varices because of the large amount of nitrogenous material pouring into the intestinal tract in the presence of demonstrable portal-systemic shunts, and the hyperammoniemia and coma represent a significant cause of death. The pathophysiology of this disorder has already been discussed. Treatment consists of vigorous catharsis and enemas to empty the gastrointestinal tract of accumulated blood, the administration of liquid neomycin in dosages of 2 gm. every four hours for the first 24 hour period and the use of ion exchange resins given by colonic instillation. The use of these resins is attended by considerable potassium depletion, and the added sodium they will provide for the total body stores is likely to increase the problem of accumulating ascites. The amino acids (L-glutamic acid and L-arginine) have been utilized in the form of a salt for intravenous administration in hepatic encephalopathy. Glutamic acid has been well demonstrated to be both metabolically and clinically effective, but the action of this amino acid in binding ammonia to form glutamine is reversible, and only temporary improvement can be anticipated unless the source of the ammonia formation is corrected. Arginine in theory would be effective by providing further substrate for the cycle of urea synthesis; while clinical effectiveness has been suggested in some studies, there are no supportive metabolic data to indicate that this affects the syndrome of ammonia intoxication to any significant degree. (See Chapter 4 for a more detailed discussion of the clinical and metabolic effects of L-glutamic acid and L-arginine.) Since the syndrome of ammonia intoxication is usually reversible if the bleeding can be controlled, it is ordinarily unnecessary to consider more drastic measures such as exchange transfusion or dialysis in the treatment of this particular metabolic abnormality. It should be emphasized that this type of encephalopathy is common even in patients with well compensated cirrhosis since it is dependent on shunting and decrease in hepatic blood flow rather than on a primary hepatocellular defect.

Ascites will very commonly appear in association with episodes of bleeding varices. Even when there is not pre-existing ascites, the existence of some degree of intrahepatic portal bed block and a defect in albumin synthesis will make these individuals extremely liable to the accumulation of ascitic fluid if any significant degree of salt retention occurs. The hypovolemia that is inevitable with any severe degree of bleeding induces an adrenal response with hyperaldosteronism; the stage is set for sodium and water retention and accompanying ascites. It is therefore important not to provide any added salt in administered intravenous fluids. Once bleeding is controlled, this ascites will usually dissipate spontaneously over a period of several days, but it may provide an added metabolic problem if abdominal surgery of any kind becomes indicated. Under these circumstances, one can anticipate a reaccumulation of ascites in the immediate postoperative period requiring administration of adequate amounts of plasma or human serum albumin or both.

Abnormal liver function is of course inevitable with intrahepatic portal bed block from cirrhosis but varies considerably in degree in the patients with bleeding esophageal varices. If liver reserve is very seriously impaired before the bleeding episode, the hemorrhage and attendant problems already described will inevitably result in further deterioration in hepatic cell function so that fulminant and progressive liver failure may ensue. Under these circumstances, this is almost inexorably fatal, but the details of possible methods of management have been discussed in the section concerned with hepatic encephalopathy and fulminant hepatic failure.

If the episode of bleeding from esophageal varices is controlled without construction of an urgent shunt, the surgeon must then consider the advisability and timing of more definitive surgery for portal hypertension. This problem will be reviewed in a subsequent chapter on elective shunts.

bibliography

Belkin, G. A., and Conn, H. O.: Blood ammonia concentration and bromsulfalein retention in upper gastrointestinal hemorrhage. New Eng. J. Med., *260:*530–534, 1959.

Bennett, H. D., Baker, L., and Baker, L. A.: Complications in the use of esophageal compression balloons (Sengstaken tube). Arch. Int. Med., *90:*196–200, 1952.

Britton, R. C., and Crile, G., Jr.: Late results of transesophageal suture of bleeding esophageal varices. Surg. Gynec. Obstet., *117:*10–14, 1963.

Conn, H. F.: Bleeding esophageal varices. *In* Conn, H. F. (Ed.): Current Therapy. Philadelphia, W. B. Saunders Co., 1965, pp. 245–247.

Conn, H. O.: Hazards attending the use of esophageal tamponade. New Eng. J. Med., *259:*701–707, 1958.

Conn, H. O.: Excessive mortality associated with balloon tamponade of bleeding varices. A critical reappraisal. J. A. M. A., *202:*587–591, 1967.

Conn, H. O., and Brodoff, M.: Emergency esophagoscopy in the diagnosis of upper gastrointestinal hemorrhage. A critical evaluation of its diagnostic accuracy. Gastroenterology, *47:*505-512, 1964.

Conn, H. O., and Dalessio, D. J.: Multiple infusions of posterior pituitary extract in the treatment of bleeding esophageal varices. Ann. Int. Med., *57:*804-809, 1962.

Conn, H. O., Mitchell, J. R., and Brodoff, M. G.: A comparison of the radiologic and esophagoscopic diagnosis of esophageal varices. New Eng. J. Med., *265:*160-164, 1961.

Conn, H. O., Smith, H. W., and Brodoff, M.: Observer variation in the endoscopic diagnosis of esophageal varices. A prospective investigation of the diagnostic validity of esophagoscopy. New Eng. J. Med., *272:* 830-834, 1965.

Dagradi, A., Sanders, D., and Stempien, J.: The sources of upper gastrointestinal bleeding in liver cirrhosis. Ann. Int. Med., *42:*852-855, 1955.

Eckman, C.-A., and Sandblom, P.: Shunt operation in acute bleeding from esophageal varicosities. Ann. Surg., *160:*531-539, 1964.

Kirsh, I. E., Blackwell, C. C., and Bennett, H. D.: Roentgen diagnosis of esophageal varices. Comparison of roentgen and esophagoscopic findings in 502 cases. Amer. J. Roentgen., *74:*477-485, 1955.

Linton, R. R., and Ellis, D. S.: Emergency and definitive treatment of bleeding esophageal varices. J. A. M. A., *160:*1017-1023, 1956.

Mackby, M. J.: Treatment of bleeding esophageal varices. J. A. M. A., *171:*1916-1922, 1959.

McDermott, W. V., Jr.: A simple discriminatory test for upper gastrointestinal hemorrhage. New Eng. J. Med., *257:*1161-1164, 1957.

McDermott, W. V., Jr.: The management of bleeding esophageal varices. Med. Sci. *16:*51-57, 1965.

McDermott, W. V., Jr.: Bleeding esophageal varices. *In* Conn, H. F. (Ed.): Current Therapy. Philadelphia, W. B. Saunders Co., 1968, pp. 287-288.

McDermott, W. V., Jr., Wareham, J., and Riddell, A. G.: Treatment of "hepatic coma" with L-glutamic acid. New Eng. J. Med., *253:*1093-1102, 1955.

McDermott, W. V., Jr., Wareham, J., and Riddell, A. G.: Bleeding esophageal varices. A study of the cause of the associated "hepatic coma." Ann. Surg., *144:*318-335, 1956.

Merigan, T. C., Jr., et al.: Gastrointestinal bleeding with cirrhosis. A study of 172 episodes in 158 patients. New Eng. J. Med., *263:*579-585, 1960.

Mikkelsen, W. P.: Emergency portacaval shunt. Rev. Surg. (Phila.), *19:*141-148, 1962.

Nachlas, M. M., O'Neill, J. E., and Campbell, A. J. A.: The life history of patients with cirrhosis of the liver and bleeding esophageal varices. Ann. Surg., *141:*10-23, 1955.

Nusbaum, M., Baum, S., and Blakemore, W. S.: Clinical experience with the diagnosis and management of gastrointestinal hemorrhage by selective mesenteric catheterization. Ann. Surg., *170:*506-514, 1969.

Orloff, M. J.: Emergency portacaval shunt: A comparative study of shunt, varix ligation and nonsurgical treatment of bleeding esophageal varices in unselected patients with cirrhosis. Ann. Surg., *166:*456-478, 1967.

Palmer, E. D.: On the natural history of esophageal varices which are secondary to portal cirrhosis. Ann. Int. Med., *47:*18-26, 1957.

Panke, W. F., Rousselot, L. M., and Moreno, A. H.: Splenic pulp manometry as an emergency test in the differential diagnosis of acute upper gastrointestinal bleeding. Surg. Gynec. Obstet., *109:*270-278, 1959.

Rousselot, L. M., Gilbertson, F. E., and Panke, W. F.: Severe hemorrhage from esophagogastric varices. Its emergency management with particular reference to portacaval anastomosis. New Eng. J. Med., *262:*269–276, 1960.

Rousselot, L. M., Moreno, A. H., and Panke, W. F.: Studies on portal hypertension. IV. The clinical and physiopathologic significance of self-established (nonsurgical) portal systemic venous shunts. Ann. Surg., *150:*384–412, 1959.

Sengstaken, R. W., and Blakemore, A. H.: Balloon tamponade for the control of hemorrhage from esophageal varices. Ann. Surg., *131:*781–789, 1950.

Turner, M. D., Sherlock, S., and Steiner, R. E.: Splenic venography and intrasplenic pressure measurement in the clinical investigation of the portal venous system. Amer. J. Med., *23:*846–859, 1957.

Warthin, T. A., Ross, F. P., Baker, D. V., Jr., and Wissing, E.: The management of upper gastrointestinal hemorrhage. Ann. Int. Med., *39:*241–253, 1953.

Weinberger, H. A.: Emergency portacaval shunt for esophagogastric hemorrhage. Arch. Surg., *91:*333–337, 1965.

Weinberger, H. A., and Maier, H. C.: Early portacaval shunt in selected cases of massive hemorrhage from esophageal varices. Surgery, *49:*707–712, 1961.

Welch, C. S., et al.: Treatment of bleeding from portal hypertension in patients with cirrhosis of the liver. New Eng. J. Med., *254:*493–502, 1956.

Zamcheck, N., et al.: Early roentgen diagnosis in massive bleeding from the upper gastrointestinal tract. I. Clinical evaluation of safety and reliability of the method in 123 patients. Amer. J. Med., *13:*713–724, 1952.

Elective Shunts and Other Procedures in the Treatment of Portal Hypertension

CHAPTER 7

In 1877 Eck demonstrated that the construction of a shunt between the portal and systemic circulation was compatible with survival in the dog. After that, a number of similar procedures were carried out in experimental animals in order to study the general effects of this procedure. Over the subsequent years, a few sporadic attempts were made to utilize this operative procedure in man for the control of either ascites or hemorrhage, but none of these was followed by any long term survivals. Whipple in 1945 and Blakemore in 1947 reported the initial results of their directed surgical approach to the problems of portal hypertension. Over the subsequent years, various operations to achieve portal-systemic shunting came into wide usage, and numbers of clinical and experimental studies directed toward this particular problem have been reported by us and many others in order to evaluate the present role of portal-systemic shunts and to analyze the results of these procedures in terms of control of hemorrhage or ascites, immediate early mortality and long term survival and post-shunt complications such as encephalopathy and peptic ulceration.

types of shunts

In Figure 7-1 various types of portal-systemic shunts in fairly common usage are shown diagrammatically. A number of so-called makeshift shunts have been reported over the years; the variety and relative rarity of these make any rational analysis impossible and they

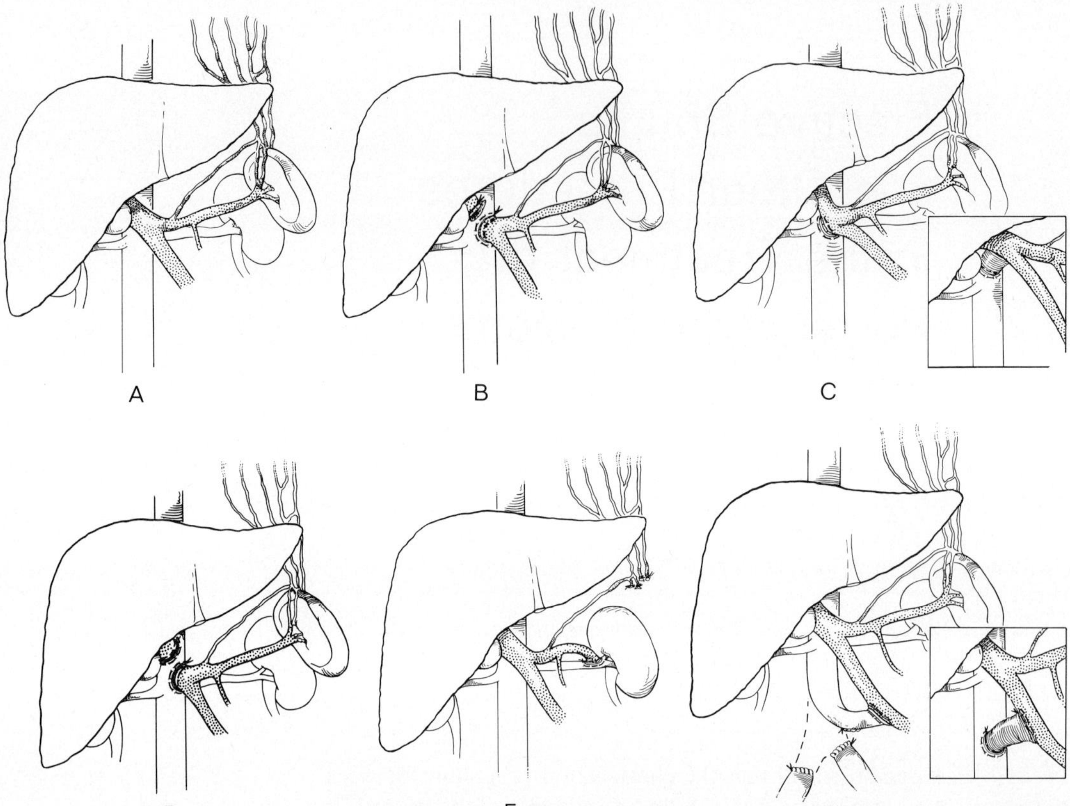

A B C D E F

FIG. 7-1. Common types of portal-systemic shunts: A, Venous anatomy in portal hypertension. B, End-to-side portacaval shunt. C, Side-to-side portacaval shunt (insert—with synthetic graft). D, Double portacaval shunt. E, Splenorenal shunt. F, Mesocaval shunt (insert—with graft.)

are not included in this survey. It is important to note in this diagram that every one of the shunts, except for the end-to-side portacaval, provides a potential route of reverse flow from the intrahepatic circulation through and into the systemic circulation. In other words, except for the direct end-to-side portacaval shunt, in which the hepatic side of the divided portal vein is ligated, all the other procedures shown are similar from the hemodynamic or physiologic point of view to a side-to-side portacaval shunt, although the degree of decompression accomplished depends on a number of factors such as pressure, flow and actual size of the shunt that it is possible to construct.

The techniques of constructing these shunts and the hemodynamic changes associated with portal-systemic shunting are covered in other sections, and attention will be directed in this chapter towards the clinical results and complications.

In Table 7-1, we have summarized a number of series of portal-systemic shunts that emphasize some of the major aspects of the surgical problem. Obviously, these data do not provide a simple answer to the complexities of the problem. Various aspects of the clinical evaluation of shunting will be taken up individually. It is also important to realize that the patient material varies in each series and that the admixture of types of shunts makes valid comparisons difficult. In addition, since many of the series reported stretch over a number of years, a great many factors that are very difficult to define will go into a single simple figure reported as a percentage. Despite the range, there are certain interesting similarities that occur in this table. The hospital mortality for elective portal-systemic shunting is in the general range of 10 per cent. The effectiveness of shunts in terms of control of bleeding seems quite definite since over 85 per cent of the patients have no further bleeding from esophageal varices. This figure will vary widely, however, since different types of shunts in various proportions have been utilized by the reporting surgeons. The five year survival is reasonably consistent and is in the range of 50 per cent. Postshunt encephalopathy is obviously a serious complication of this surgical procedure, and it would be fair to say that about 25 per cent of all patients who have had shunts constructed develop some neuropsychiatric manifestations. Again, this percentage will vary with the type of shunt, the selection of patients and the meticulousness with which this complication is sought for and observed. Peptic ulceration is a less frequent problem after shunt surgery, but most authors have recognized this as occurring in roughly 10 per cent of patients. Again, in this chapter, the problem of postshunt encephalopathy will be reviewed, but many of the details of

TABLE 7-1. Elective Portal-Systemic Shunts

Author	Dates	Hospital Mortality (%)	Incidence of Rebleeding from Varices (%)	5 Year Survival (%)	Postshunt Encephalopathy (%)	Peptic Ulcer (%)
McDermott	1961	9	15	68	18	15
Walker	1961	6	12	70	20	—
Sedgwick	1966	21.5	21.2	57.1	22.5	5
Child	1956	14	—	—	—	—
Palmer	1957	10.5	14	—	—	—
Foster	1971	19	10	40	19	4
Akkary (schistosomiasis)	1962	23	10	—	26	—
Zuidema	1961	20	—	—	15	—
Schwartz	1968	5	—	47	30	—
Barnes	1971	9	14	—	—	—
Patton	1959	19	—	—	3	8
Ellis	1956	11	14.9	50	—	—
Welch	1957	15	20	—	—	—
Wantz	1961	11.3	—	—	21.8	—
Voorhees	1970	12	3	37	34	12

the pathophysiology will be covered in more detail in the sections on hemodynamics and hepatic coma.

indications for shunting

Although Eck first carried out his portacaval shunt in dogs with the concept that this might be applicable to problems of ascites in man, the introduction of this procedure into wide clinical usage by Whipple was directed primarily towards the problem of bleeding esophageal varices. Since most unselected series of patients with massive hemorrhage from esophageal varices have shown mortalities of greater than 50 per cent (in competent hands any of the ordinary types of shunts carries a hospital mortality of about 10 per cent and an incidence of rebleeding from varices of only about 10 per cent), a logical initial supposition would be that this obvious effectiveness in control of hemorrhage would prolong the lives of large numbers of patients with portal hypertension. The early studies emphasize this fact, but the mistake was often made of comparing the long term results in patients with surgical shunts with unselected series of medically managed patients, most of whom showed a mortality of 50 per cent within the first year. This did not take into account, however, the fact that surgically treated patients were obviously selected from among the better risks in the overall group of patients with this dangerous disease. Although questions were raised intermittently about the actual survival value of the shunt, it has been generally accepted for the past 25 years that any patient who represented a reasonable operative risk and who had demonstrable bleeding from esophageal varices should have some type of a portal-systemic shunt established. In a more specific discussion toward the end of this chapter, we will question this premise, although not in terms of the well established protection that an adequate shunt will give against further bleeding. In Table 7-2 are shown our data on a group of patients who have been carefully followed over more than three years. Obviously, the incidence of late postshunt bleeding is low and would support the data of others that an open and functioning portal-systemic shunt does, in fact, provide a high degree of protection against further bleeding of any type and particularly from esophageal varices.

In this light, the question then arises whether a shunt should be carried out immediately or as an elective procedure some time after the hemorrhage has been controlled. As we stated earlier, we prefer the term "urgent shunt" rather than "emergency shunt" since it is our practice to construct a shunt on a patient who enters with active bleeding only after the bleeding has been brought under control by any one of a number of nonsurgical approaches, the gut has been thoroughly cleansed of blood, the urine output well established, blood volume restored, encephalopathy corrected and the patient brought to the optimal condition under the circumstances. Ordinarily, this will

TABLE 7-2. Occurrence, Source and Outcome of Late Postshunt Bleeding

	Portacaval	Splenorenal	Total
Total discharges from hospital	52	129	181
Postshunt bleeding	8 (15%)	33 (26%)	41 (23%)
Source of bleeding:			
Esophageal varices	5 (10%)	23 (18%)	28 (15%)
Peptic ulcer	1 (2%)	5 (4%)	6 (3%)
Gastritis	1 (2%)	0	1 (0.6%)
Unknown and miscellaneous	1 (2%)	5 (4%)	6 (3%)
Death from hemorrhage	3 (6%)	12 (9%)	15 (8%)
Further surgery required:			
Additional shunt or ligation	0	10 (8%)	10 (6%)
Other	0	0	0

take from 12 to 48 hours, and thus the procedure is not truly in the category of an emergency operation. The use of the urgent shunt has been discussed in more detail in the section on the management of acute hemorrhage from esophageal varices; here we will only emphasize that we utilize this approach only under the circumstances described above and limit it to patients categorized as good risks by our own liver index calculation and by the commonly used Child classification.

Most patients will be given a trial of nonsurgical management, and if bleeding does not continue or recur, an elective shunt will be planned, selection of the type to be guided by the criteria defined in more detail later.

In the early days of shunt surgery, a patient with *ascites* was considered by Linton and others to be a poor operative risk, and, in general, ascites was felt to be a contraindication to shunt surgery. Over the subsequent years, better understanding of the pathophysiology of cirrhotic ascites has been achieved, the hemodynamic importance of the "outflow block" has been recognized, and clinical reports by Welch and by us have demonstrated that any type of shunt providing adequate decompression of both the splanchnic and intrahepatic vascular beds has been extremely effective in controlling ascites. Because of improved medical management, the presence of ascites alone is no longer a frequent indication for shunt surgery since the selected group of patients who could be subjected to surgery without an inordinate mortality can usually be ultimately controlled by medical management. However, there remain a number of patients with ascites in conjunction with bleeding esophageal varices in whom long deferment of a shunting procedure would carry a high risk of rebleeding. It is in this group primarily that the principles of combined decompression should be employed when a shunt is under consideration.

prophylactic shunts

With a mortality of greater than 50 per cent in unselected patients with their first bleed from esophageal varices, it was logical that surgeons would begin to utilize shunting as a prophylactic measure when varices appeared and before hemorrhage had occurred. Several randomized studies are now available for analysis and have, in our opinion, presented convincing evidence that, while the presence of a shunt does give a high degree of protection against variceal bleeding, the ultimate survival curve is certainly no better than that for patients managed medically. The medical group did have an increasing number of deaths from bleeding as the series was extended, but this was counterbalanced by a larger proportion of surgically treated patients who died from progressive liver failure, usually in association with encephalopathy. Thus, one must consider the quality of life in these two groups and reach a decision whether the protection against hemorrhage in the surgical group is worth the increased hepatic deterioration and absence of any increase in survival (Fig. 7-2).

therapeutic shunts

The same types of randomized studies are now in progress relative to the survival value of the shunt when it is applied therapeutically after patients have had one or more demonstrable bleeds from varices. Resnick, whose conclusions relative to the prophylactic shunt have been referred to, is directing a similar randomized study on therapeutic shunts for the Boston Inter-Hospital Liver Group. At the moment, comparative survival curves are still inconclusive although the medically treated group has had an 80 per cent incidence of rebleeding. The data reported from a similar study by Jackson and co-workers show equally conclusive data on the protection afforded by a shunt against further hemorrhage, and the survival data tend to favor the surgically treated group.

Thus, a satisfactory shunt does give a patient who has had one or more hemorrhages from esophageal varices a highly significant degree of protection against further bleeding. These studies do not, however, compare various types of operative management nor do they contribute to the identification of the high risk patients. It is important to scrutinize the complications of shunting procedures in detail with a view to providing more flexibility in the choice of surgical procedures.

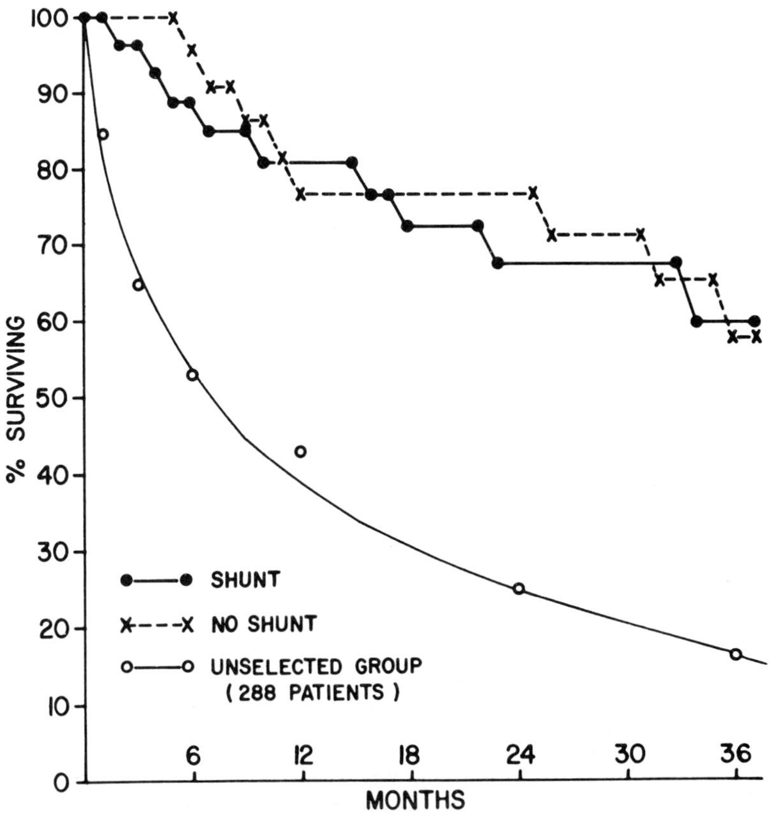

FIG. 7-2. Survival curves in the randomized prophylactic shunt study group as compared with 288 unselected patients with varices without hemorrhage. (Reproduced from Garceau, A. J., et al.: A Controlled Trial of Prophylactic Portacaval-Shunt Surgery. N. Eng. J. Med. *270*:496–500, 1964, with permission of the Publishers)

complications

Any shunting procedure is attended by the ordinary pulmonary, wound, urinary tract, cardiac and other problems associated with any major operation. In this section we will refer only to those complications that are specific for shunt constructions.

Postshunt encephalopathy is certainly the most distressing of the specific complications encountered after this type of surgery. Our own experience has been reported recently and is shown in Table 7-3. The overall incidence of 18 per cent (26 per cent in the portacaval group) is distressing, but it must be recognized that in only about 10 per cent of cases was the encephalopathy serious and incapacitating; the remainder proved to be quite easy to control with protein restriction, catharsis, lactulose or continuous or intermittent administration of intestinal antibiotics.

Those patients who are seriously affected by intractable encepha-

TABLE 7-3. Incidence of Postshunt Encephalopathy

	Total	Portacaval	Splenorenal
Shunts 1945–65	407	171	236
Encephalopathy	75 (18%)	45 (26%)	30 (12%)

lopathy do present an extremely pathetic and distressing problem. The neuropsychiatric manifestations of this problem are protean. Ordinarily, the clinical picture is one of depressed mentation with slurred speech, asterixis, varying degrees of disorientation and staggering gait; not infrequently, however, one encounters choreoathetosis, generalized or jacksonian seizures, cerebellar signs and symptoms and other less dramatic neurologic findings. This neuropsychiatric disorder and the accompanying biochemical changes have been discussed in more detail in a preceding section. Hyperammoniemia related to the amount of protein ingested is the common accompaniment of this clinical syndrome and has been generally accepted as a major metabolic abnormality and probably an etiologic factor.

For years the reason for the occurrence of this disorder in certain individuals was obscure. Certainly it was not related to classification of risk although it was certainly age related as is shown in Figure 7-3. In fact, some of the best operative risks develop the worst problems in both encephalopathy and hepatic deterioration after surgery. Some years ago, it was clinically recognized by surgeons in the Middle

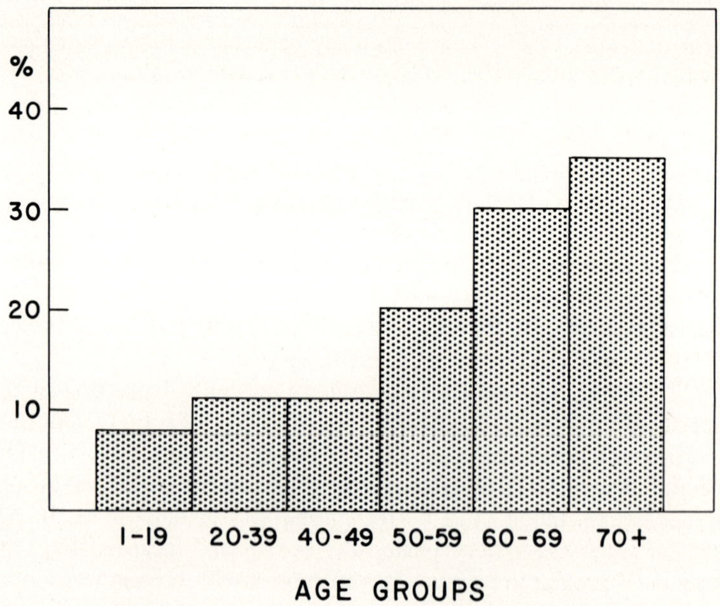

FIG. 7-3. Relationship of age to postshunt encephalopathy. (Reproduced from McDermott, W. V., Jr., et al.: Postshunt Encephalopathy. Surg. Gynec. Obstet. *126*:585–590, 1968, with permission of the Publishers)

East, Brazil and other areas where schistosomiasis is endemic that patients with this particular type of portal hypertension did not do well after shunt surgery. Studies over the recent years by Warren and Zeppa and by others have pointed up the fact that patients with a high degree of hepatofugal flow still existing in the portal vein will probably do badly after a diverting shunt. Our own data, described in the chapter on portal hemodynamics and pathophysiology, indicate that it is those patients who show a decrease in total effective hepatic blood flow after surgery who are most likely to develop severe encephalopathy and often concomitant progressive hepatic deterioration. These observations do not help, however, in predicting the patients who will do poorly. In the discussion of portal hemodynamics, we have presented data that may provide a clue to this type of identification. In the series described there, postshunt encephalopathy occurred in 53 per cent of patients in whom the difference between the free portal pressure and hepatic occluded portal pressure was greater than 10 cm. of saline; in those with relatively little change (less than 5 cm.) the incidence was 19 per cent. Presumably those in the latter group have gradually compensated for progressive decrease in flow to the liver through the portal vein. These observations will probably have increasing effect in influencing surgeons towards a better choice of operative procedures for bleeding esophageal varices, and this will be considered later in this section. Details of the management of this major complication of shunt surgery have been described in the chapter specifically concerned with encephalopathy.

peptic ulcer

Peptic ulcer has occurred in varying incidence in many of the series reported (Table 7-1). In our own patients who have been followed adequately for more than one year, the incidence has been 15 per cent, and with more recognition of this possibility, the incidence seems to be increasing. The true relationship between peptic ulcer and portacaval shunt in man has not been well established as yet, and some have questioned whether the incidence is higher than one would expect in a similar group of patients without liver disease or shunt surgery in the general population. In Orloff's studies, the incidence of peptic ulcer in cirrhotic patients without shunts was 12 per cent as contrasted with 27 per cent in a group of shunted cirrhotic patients. Of the 14 patients with peptic ulceration after shunt surgery, however, 12 had superficial erosions of the acute "stress" type such as may be encountered after any serious illness or major surgical procedure. In short, the results of a number of retrospective clinical studies relative to the actual incidence of postshunt peptic ulcer are still inconclusive, with occurrence rates ranging from 1.7 to 16 per cent. The suspicion, whether valid or not, that peptic ulcer is a specific complication of portal-systemic shunting has led Silen, Eiseman, Orloff, Clarke and others to study this problem in experimental animals.

The first laboratory studies relative to the problem of portal-systemic shunting and gastric secretion were carried out in 1933 by Lebedinskhaya who reported that construction of an Eck fistula resulted in increased gastric acid secretion in dogs with Pavlov pouches. These findings were confirmed a few years later by Gerez and Weiss, but very little further work was done during the next two decades. In 1957, Dubuque and his group observed a significant rise in gastric secretion from canine Heidenheim pouches either after gradual occlusion of the portal vein or after some type of portacaval shunt. They also found an increased ulcer diathesis in the shunted animals who were given daily injections of histamine and beeswax. Subsequently, a proliferation of experimental studies, using the dog primarily as the experimental animal, was carried out to clarify the pathophysiology of this phenomenon. While some divergence developed among various groups of investigators relative to differences between shunted and normal animals in terms of basal secretion and response to histamine stimulation, there has been general agreement that a highly significant increase in gastric acid hypersecretion occurs in the shunted animal in response to an intestinal meal, and there is a susceptibility to peptic ulceration in these experimental animals. The response to an intestinal meal varies as the composition of the feeding is changed, and maximal response is obtained from protein rather than carbohydrate and fat. Since the construction of an Eck fistula is very likely to be followed by progressive deterioration in hepatic function, the work of Clarke and associates was particularly important in demonstrating that a similar hypersecretory response occurred after an intestinal meal given to animals after portacaval transposition in whom liver blood flow and liver function were maintained at near normal levels. Orloff's studies using autotransfusion and cross transfusion techniques would appear to indicate that the secretory response is caused by unmasking of the intestinal phase of gastric secretion by the hepatic bypass of a potent intestinal hormone that stimulates the parietal cells. Ingenious studies done on the effluent blood from shunts at various levels of the gastrointestinal tract would indicate that histamine is not necessarily this specific secretagogue. Postshunt hypersecretion would appear to depend on some agent released from the intestine on contact with food, but whether this substance originates from the intestine itself or from the ingested food is still unclear.

Thus, the evidence to date would appear to be incontrovertible that a powerful gastric secretagogue is released into the portal circulation after an intestinal meal and that this secretagogue is normally inactivated by the liver. Ingestion of a meal high in protein seems to be the strongest stimulating factor for this secretagogue, but a significant response has occurred after balloon distention of the small intestine. The exact nature of the humoral agent elaborated is unclear. There is conflicting evidence on the specificity of histamine, and Thompson has suggested that it may well be an intestinal form of gastrin whose active tetrapeptide fragment is in an exposed position and therefore easily deactivated as it passes through the liver.

In terms of clinical observations, Orloff's studies on gastric secretion after portacaval shunt in man would appear to be similar to those described in the experimental animal and indicate that a striking increase in gastric secretory activity does occur after the ingestion of a protein meal in patients who have had surgically constructed portacaval shunts. Whether or not this well defined responsive gastric hypersecretion is accompanied by an increase in peptic ulceration is far from clear, as already noted. Reports of highly malignant and intractable peptic ulcer occurring after shunt surgery would suggest a relationship in some instances whether or not the overall incidence is increased. Pertinent to the clinical management of these patients is the report by Filoso, Jacobson and Silen of two postshunt patients in whom hypochlorhydria had been surgically induced to treat a peptic ulcer syndrome, and severe encephalopathy occurred that had not existed prior to the gastric surgery. It was suggested by the authors that the diminished acid output and the resultant overgrowth of small bowel flora might enhance the production of ammonia.

In terms of clinical management, the surgeon should be acutely aware of the possibility of peptic ulceration occurring after the construction of portacaval shunt because this can result in a particularly serious combination of problems. If the ulcer bleeds in the presence of a patent portal-systemic shunt, acute encephalopathy is very likely to develop unless urgent measures are undertaken immediately to control the hemorrhage and to treat the impending hepatic coma. The problem becomes particularly difficult when one considers the effects of surgical operations on gastric secretion and the resultant effects of hypochlorhydria in the development of chronic encephalopathy.

hepatorenal syndrome

The occurrence of renal failure after shunt surgery is an ominous event. The various pathophysiologic disorders associated with the development of a "hepatorenal syndrome" have been covered in more detail in a previous chapter. If the onset of oliguria is caused by hypovolemia either from uncompensated blood loss or because of rapid reaccumulation of ascites, treatment with adequate amounts of blood, plasma or albumin is effective. On the other hand, the still inexplicable occurrence of renal insufficiency in patients with severe hepatocellular failure is usually irreversible even though the kidneys may show no structural changes at autopsy.

combined portal and caval hypertension

A serious problem associated with shunt surgery has only recently come to our attention although it may well have been missed over the years and conceivably could account for some of the patients who bled from esophageal varices after construction of an apparently adequate portal-systemic shunt. Within a few weeks, two patients presented with elevated caval pressures caused by partial constriction of the retrohepatic vena cava by hypertrophy of the caudate lobe. Both patients died from massive hemorrhage during the early postoperative phase after shunt surgery, and in both instances it was well documented that elevated pressure in the subhepatic vena cava prevented adequate decompression of portal hypertension. Autopsies were obtained on both patients demonstrating the mechanical constriction of the retrohepatic vena cava. Figure 7-4 illustrates the problem as seen at postmortem examination, and both case histories are summarized to illustrate the problem.

CASE 1: A 50 year old man was treated electively for recurrent bleeding from esophageal varices with an end-to-side portacaval shunt. At operation, portal pressure was 325 mm. of water. At the conclusion of the shunt construction the pressure had dropped only 40 mm. of water, and then inferior caval pressure was recorded at 285 mm. of water with a concomitant superior caval pressure of 100 mm. The patient died on the tenth postoperative day of a massive gastrointestinal hemorrhage. At postmortem examination, a hypertrophied caudate lobe was found to be constricting the lumen of the retrohepatic vena cava to a diameter of 5 mm.

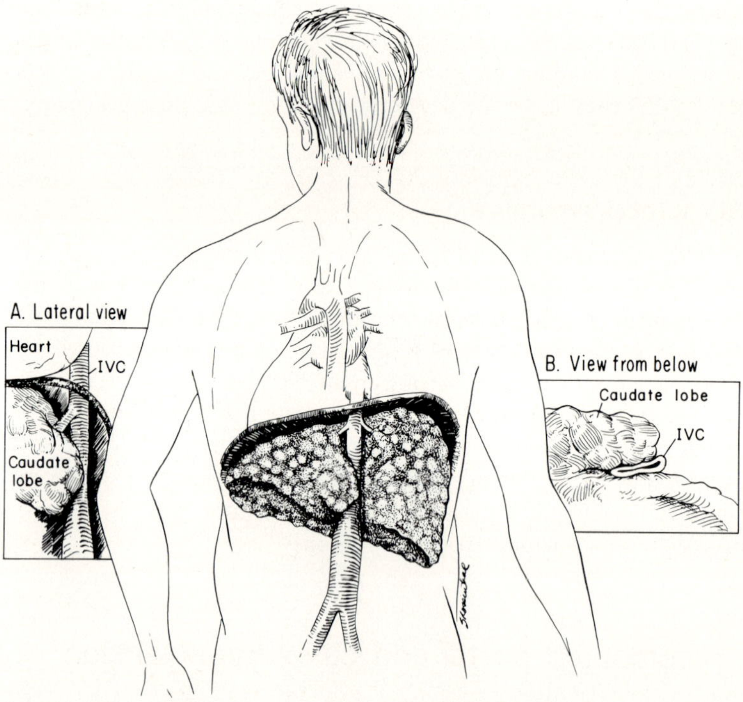

FIG. 7-4. The mechanism by which cirrhosis produced subhepatic caval hypertension in Case 1 (see text). (Reproduced from Welling, R. E., and McDermott, W. V., Jr.: Combined Caval and Portal Hypertension with Cirrhosis of the Liver: A Problem in Management. Ann. Surg., in Press, with permission of the Publishers)

CASE 2: A 40 year old man entered with massive bleeding from esophageal varices and an urgent portacaval shunt was constructed. The free portal pressure was 380 mm. of water, and the subhepatic vena caval pressure was 260 mm. Opening of the shunt resulted in a drop in pressure of only 25 mm. Bleeding continued, and the patient died on the third postoperative day. At postmortem examination the diameter of the retrohepatic vena was narrowed by 7 mm. by large regenerating nodules in the caudate lobe.

In both instances, recognition of the significant elevation of pressure in the subhepatic vena cava should have directed us away from the construction of a shunt and towards some other type of procedure such as portal-azygous disconnection as a mechanism for controlling the bleeding from esophageal varices. As a result of this experience, it is certainly recommended that after dissection of the subhepatic vena cava, manometric pressures be obtained and elevations over 200 mm. of water should probably preclude any effort towards controlling portal hypertension by shunt surgery.

choice of shunt

From both clinical data and hemodynamic evaluation of surgical procedures for portal hypertension, it is impossible to be dogmatic in terms of choice of a specific shunting procedure. In fact, it may well be that, in patients with a high degree of hepatofugal flow in the portal vein, no shunt is indicated, and a type of portal-azygous disconnection is preferable. The role of the distal and central splenorenal shunts still awaits a long term follow-up so final clinical evaluation is not possible as yet. Based on what information is available, however, each of the relatively common types of shunt will be discussed individually.

end-to-side portacaval shunt

This procedure is the most common and technically easiest procedure used in the decompression of portal hypertension. Because of the widespread experience in general surgery, utilization of this type of shunt is still probably preferable in the great majority of cases. It is, in our opinion, contraindicated in patients who have had previous right upper quadrant surgery, who have thrombocytopenia, with less than 50,000 platelets per cu.mm., or who have a large volume of ascitic fluid.

side-to-side or double portacaval shunt

Because of the high degree of combined splanchnic and hepatic decompression that is achieved with both of these shunts, they are preferable in patients who have a sufficient degree of postsinusoidal block to develop ascites. Although the double shunt is in theory more effective from a hemodynamic point of view, we have found little difference in clinical results between the two shunts in terms of postoperative dissipation of ascites. Therefore, technical considerations relative to the experience of the operator in either procedure, the size of the caudate lobe, angle between the portal vein and vena cava, distance between the two veins and ease of mobilization of a large length of portal vein would dictate which of the two should be used.

mesocaval shunt

The procedure by which the inferior vena cava (or rather, the right common iliac vein) is turned upward, brought through the mesentery of the right colon and anastomosed to the side of the superior mesenteric vein, as described originally and independently by Clatworthy and by Marion, is ideal for the patient with an extrahepatic block who has had previous splenectomy. Functionally, it acts as a side-to-side shunt. Some surgeons, Voorhees in particular, have utilized it as a procedure of choice, feeling that it is technically straightforward and relatively simple and has good clinical results. As far as can be determined, there is no discernible difference between this procedure and a side-to-side shunt from the point of view of function, so that it remains in the area of the operator's choice. Our own experience has been relatively limited, but we have encountered no serious contraindications to the procedure. If, during attempted construction of a side-to-side shunt, the portal vein, because of unanticipated thrombosis or for anatomic reasons, is not satisfactory, the operator can shift easily through the same incision and construct a mesocaval shunt. The use of a Teflon graft between the cava and the superior mesenteric veins, as described by Drapanas, may greatly simplify the technique if long term patency can be confirmed.

splenorenal shunt

Perhaps the greatest controversy in terms of choice of shunts has existed between the proponents of the splenorenal shunt and those of the portacaval shunt. Functionally, the splenorenal shunt acts as a small side-to-side shunt. While the size of the splenic vein varies considerably, it is ordinarily the smallest of the shunts in common usage, and, as might be anticipated, there is a higher incidence of rebleeding from esophageal varices either because of thrombosis of the shunt or because of inadequacy of the decompression. To balance this disadvantage, however, there is a distinctly lower incidence of postshunt encephalopathy. This puts the surgeon in the position of Odysseus sailing between Scylla and Charybdis. Our own preference is in general towards a type of portacaval shunt, but we utilize the splenorenal shunt preferentially in patients who have had previous right upper quadrant surgery, who have demonstrable extrahepatic block and, in particular, in those who have a high degree of thrombocytopenia (less than 50,000 platelets per cu.mm.).

The problem of hypersplenism and thrombocytopenia in portal hypertension is of considerable interest; presumably this is caused by sequestration and destruction of circulating blood elements in a greatly enlarged and congested spleen. The contention that adequate decompression of portal hypertension will bring about a resolution of the hypersplenism is not borne out by fact. In our own experience, only about 50 per cent of patients who have some combination of anemia, leukopenia and thrombocytopenia will improve after a portacaval shunt, whereas splenectomy will invariably correct this hematologic abnormality. In Rousselot's experience, recognition of this inadequacy of the portacaval shunt led him to carry out splenectomy after the construction of the shunt, but if the splenic vein is adequate (greater than 1.0 cm. in diameter by splenoportography), we feel that a splenorenal shunt is the procedure of choice. If this particular shunt is elected, intravenous pyelography should always be part of the preoperative workup since absence of the left kidney or damage at the time of operation to a solitary left kidney would be a surgical disaster.

renoportal shunt

This procedure (Fig. 7-5) was introduced to circumvent some of the difficult technical problems that may be encountered in the attempt to approximate the portal vein and the vena cava for a lateral anastomosis. Functionally, it is similar to a side-to-side portacaval shunt, and interruption of the left renal vein at that distance from the kidney has not caused any impairment of function.

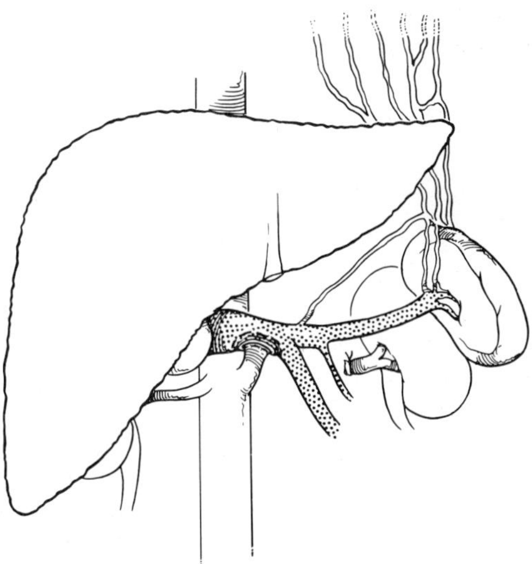

FIG. 7-5. Renoportal shunt

central splenorenal and distal splenorenal shunts

The possible utilization of these procedures as designed by Warren and by Britton has been discussed in the section on hemodynamics. Both of these procedures may be technically difficult for the surgeon without experience in this area; both are designed to provide some degree of portal decompression without diverting portal blood flow from the liver. At the present time one cannot comment on these ingenious approaches to portal hypertension since long term clinical results are not available.

portacaval or renoportal transposition (Fig. 7-6)

Reference has been made in several sections of this book to the fact that maintenance of blood flow to the liver in the experimental animal by either portacaval or portarenal transposition will almost totally negate the adverse effects of the standard Eck fistula in terms of protection against hyperammoniemia, postshunt encephalopathy and progressive hepatic and metabolic deterioration. One could reasonably ask why this procedure has not been applied in man. One of the obvious problems involves technical difficulties; without the use of intervening synthetic or autogenous grafts it frequently would be impossible to join the divided ends of the portal vein and the subhepatic vena cava. In one instance, we were able to accomplish this procedure with some difficulty, but because of factors not related to the technical procedure itself, the patient died. There is no question, however, that in most instances the enlargement of the liver, hypertrophy of the caudate lobe, distortion of the normal anatomy that results from cirrhosis and portal hypertension would preclude the construction of a satisfactory portacaval transposition. When it became apparent that renoportal transposition was technically easier and metabolically a very satisfactory procedure in the dog, this operation was carried out on one patient in this department (Fig. 7-6B). Imme-

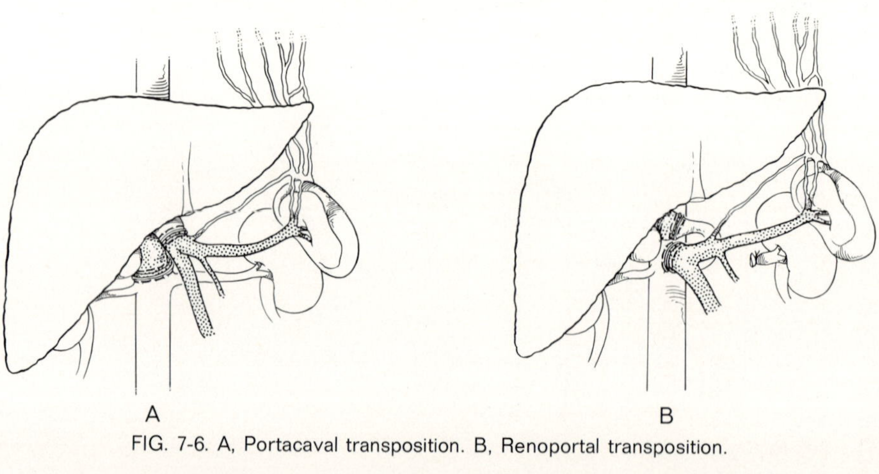

FIG. 7-6. A, Portacaval transposition. B, Renoportal transposition.

diately after this operation was completed, it was obvious that the flow through the anastomosis between the divided renal vein and the hepatic end of the divided portal vein was not in the direction of the liver but rather from the liver in a retrograde fashion into a congested kidney with the effluent blood presumably being carried off by collateral venous channels surrounding the kidney itself. At any rate, it was clear that in the presence of a high degree of portal bed block, relatively low venous pressure could not be expected to perfuse the liver adequately and that no effective maintenance of flow would be accomplished. In fact, this particular patient promptly developed chronic recurrent postshunt encephalopathy after operation.

It would appear, therefore, that the combination of considerable technical difficulty in constructing some type of transposition and the unlikelihood that prograde flow could be achieved in the presence of any significant degree of intrahepatic portal bed block makes it seem highly unlikely that this procedure would ever be applicable to most of the clinical problems of portal hypertension in man.

miscellaneous procedures

In an effort to avoid some of the metabolic problems associated with almost any type of shunting procedure, various other operations have been devised to control recurrent bleeding from esophageal varices.

TRANSTHORACIC LIGATION OF ESOPHAGEAL VARICES. Most surgeons limit the use of this procedure to controlling active bleeding from esophageal varices. Crile, however, has advocated this as a definitive procedure, particularly in the child, and has reported some good long term results. In general, however, in the adult with extrahepatic block, one can anticipate only a respite of a few weeks to a few months before bleeding will recur regardless of how thoroughly the varices have been oversewn. Ordinarily this procedure is carried out through the chest, but as described by Welch some years ago, it may be done through an abdominal approach although the hard and enlarged left lobe of the cirrhotic liver decreases accessibility to the cardioesophageal junction from the transgastric route.

PORTAL AZYGOUS DISCONNECTION. This operation, which consists of ligation of the coronary vein and the vasa brevia and transection with reanastomosis of the upper stomach, has been advocated for some years by Tanner and is often referred to by this eponym. He has reported a 20 per cent incidence of rebleeding in early reports, which is higher than one finds in any type of satisfactory shunt, but, on the other hand, the metabolic problems associated with a shunt can be avoided. This is probably the procedure of choice at the moment in most cases of schistosomiasis and may well be preferable in other patients with presinusoidal type of block in whom the portal vein still carries a significant proportion of the total liver blood flow. Many surgeons combine this with splenectomy although this will prevent subsequent usage of the splenic vein for a shunt.

PERIESOPHAGEAL STRIPPING AND PERIESOPHAGEAL LIGATION. This operation consists of a long and tedious dissection and ligation of all the veins feeding from the congested portal circulation into the area of the upper stomach, cardioesophageal junction and esophagus. Allison has been the primary advocate of this procedure, but it has never achieved widespread usage.

TRANSPOSITION OF THE SPLEEN. As described by Turinen, this consists of mobilization of the spleen through a thoracic or thoracoabdominal incision, transposition into the left chest, closure of the diaphragm around the hilar vessels and fixation of the transposed spleen into an open segment of the left lower lobe. Conceptually, this is designed to provide collateral circulation from the spleen to the pulmonary veins. As a treatment for varices, the incidence of immediate and late bleeding has been high in small series reported. Recently, Strauch has reported an extremely satisfactory result from this procedure in the treatment of Chiari syndrome in a child; this may prove to be the major usefulness of the procedure.

OTHERS. The Talma-Morison omentopexy, abrasion of the surface of the liver that abuts the diaphragm, multiple arterial ligations and several other procedures are now of historic interest only since they probably will provide no satisfactory solution to any of the problems of portal hypertension.

summary

An attempt has been made to summarize the present status of shunt surgery for portal hypertension, to identify the complications directly related to shunting procedures and to outline, as rationally as the inadequate evidence at the present time permits, the reasons that may dictate to the operating surgeon the choice of a particular type of shunt. The degree of controversy that exists in this area is obvious testimony to the fact that no one procedure is suited to all patients with portal hypertension and that further hemodynamic studies and categorization of patients are necessary before a thoroughly rational and logical choice can be made in each individual instance.

bibliography

general

Akkary, S., and Badawi, H.: The results of porta-caval shunt operation in the treatment of bleeding gastro-oesophageal varices, secondary to bilharzial hepatic fibrosis. Alexandria Med. J., *8*:338–347, 1962.

Baker, L. A., Smith, C., and Lieberman, G.: The natural history of esophageal varices. A study of 115 cirrhotic patients in whom varices were diagnosed prior to bleeding. Amer. J. Med., *26:*228-237, 1959.

Barnes, B. A., et al.: Elective portasystemic shunts: morbidity and survival data. Ann. Surg., *174:*76-84, 1971.

Blakemore, A. H.: Portacaval shunt for portal hypertension. Follow-up results in cases of cirrhosis of the liver. J. A. M. A., *145:*1335-1339, 1951.

Britton, R. C., and Crile, G., Jr.: Late results of transesophageal suture of bleeding esophageal varices. Surg. Gynec. Obstet., *117:*10-14, 1963.

Child, C. G., III: Present status of portal decompression for portal hypertension. Amer. J. Gastroent., *25:*148-153, 1956.

Child, C. G., III: The Liver and Portal Hypertension. Philadelphia, W. B. Saunders Co., 1964, p. 50.

Conn, H. O., and Lindenmuth, W. W.: Prophylactic portacaval anastomosis in cirrhotic patients with esophageal varices. A preliminary report of a controlled study. New Eng. J. Med., *266:*743-749, 1962.

Conn, H. O., and Lindenmuth, W. W.: Prophylactic portacaval anastomosis in cirrhotic patients with esophageal varices. A progress report of a continuing study. New Eng. J. Med., *272:*1255-1263, 1965.

Conn, H. O., and Lindenmuth, W. W.: Prophylactic portacaval anastomosis in cirrhotic patients with esophageal varices. Interim results, with suggestions for subsequent investigations. New Eng. J. Med., *279:*725-732, 1968.

Conn, H. O., and Lindenmuth, W. W.: Prophylactic portacaval anastomosis in cirrhotic patients with esophageal varices and ascites. Experimental design and preliminary results. Amer. J. Surg., *117:*656-661, 1969.

Drapanas, T.: Interposition mesocaval shunt for treatment of portal hypertension. Ann. Surg., *176:*435-448, 1972.

Ellis, D. S., Linton, R. R., and Jones, C. M.: Effect of venous-shunt surgery on liver function in patients with portal hypertension. A follow-up study of 125 patients operated on in the last ten years. New Eng. J. Med., *254:*931-936, 1956.

Garceau, A. J., et al.: A controlled trial of prophylactic portacaval-shunt surgery. New Eng. J. Med., *270:*496-500, 1964.

Grace, N. D., Muench, H., and Chalmers, T. C.: The present status of shunts for portal hypertension in cirrhosis. Gastroenterology, *50:*684-691, 1966.

Hallenbeck, G. A., Wollaeger, E. E., Adson, M. A., and Gage, R. P.: Results after portal-systemic shunts in 120 patients with cirrhosis of the liver. Surg. Gynec. Obstet., *116:*435-442, 1963.

Hermann, R. E., and Taylor, P. C.: The results of selection of patients for portal-systemic shunt. Surg. Gynec. Obstet., *133:*1008-1012, 1971.

Jackson, F. C., Perrin, E. B., Felix, W. R., and Smith, A. G.: A clinical investigation of the portacaval shunt: V. Survival analysis of the therapeutic operation. Ann. Surg., *174:*672-701, 1971.

King, H., and Shumacker, H. B., Jr.: Venous shunt procedures for portal hypertension in children. Surgery, *43:*680-682, 1958.

Large, A., Johnston, C. G., and Preshaw, D. E.: The portacaval venous shunt. With special reference to side-to-side portacaval anastomosis. Ann. Surg., *135:*22-33, 1952.

Linton, R. R.: Portacaval shunts in the treatment of portal hypertension. With special reference to patients previously operated upon. New Eng. J. Med., *238:*723-727, 1948.

Linton, R. R.: The surgical treatment of bleeding esophageal varices by portal systemic venous shunts with a report of 34 cases. Ann. Int. Med., *31:*794–804, 1949.

Linton, R. R.: The selection of patients for portacaval shunts. With a summary of the results in 61 cases. Ann. Surg., *134:*433–443, 1951.

Malt, R. A.: Control of massive upper gastrointestinal hemorrhage. New Eng. J. Med., *286:*1043–1046, 1972.

McDermott, W. V., Jr., Pikula, J. V., and Brown, H.: Surgery of the liver. Gastroenterology *53:*778–789, 1967.

McDermott, W. V., Jr., Palazzi, H., Nardi, G. L. and Mondet, A.: Elective portal systemic shunt. An analysis of 237 cases. New Eng. J. Med., *264:*419–427, 1961.

Nachlas, M. M.: A critical evaluation of venous shunts for the treatment of cirrhotic patients with esophageal varices. Ann. Surg., *148:*169–183, 1958.

Orloff, M. J.: Emergency portacaval shunt: A comparative study of shunt, varix ligation and nonsurgical treatment of bleeding esophageal varices in unselected patients with cirrhosis. Ann. Surg., *166:*456–478, 1967.

Palmer, E. D., Jahnke, E. J., Jr., and Hughes, C. W.: Evaluation of clinical results of portal decompression in cirrhosis. J. A. M. A. *164:*746–748, 1957.

Resnick, R. H.: The prophylactic portacaval shunt. An examination of "clinical judgment." Med. Times, *98:*93–103, 1970.

Palmer, E. D.: Personal communication, 1972.

Palmer, E. D., et al.: A controlled study of the prophylactic portacaval shunt. A final report. Ann. Int. Med., *70:*675–688, 1969.

Resnicoff, S. A., and Schwartz, S. I.: Portal decompression surgery. Comparative evaluation of patients with Laennec's cirrhosis and other causes. Arch. Surg., *97:*371–379, 1968.

Reynolds, T. B., et al.: Clinical comparison of end-to-side and side-to-side portacaval shunt. New Eng. J. Med., *274:*706–710, 1966.

Riddell, A. G., Bloor, K., Hobbs, K. E. F., and Jacquet, N.: Elective splenorenal anastomosis. Brit. Med. J., *1:*731–732, 1972.

Rousselot, L. M., Panke, W. F., Bono, R. F., and Moreno, A. H.: Experiences with portacaval anastomosis. Analysis of 104 elective end-to-side shunts for the prevention of recurrent hemorrhage from esophagogastric varices (1952 through 1961). Amer. J. Med., *34:*297–307, 1963.

Sedgwick, C. E., Poulantzas, J. K., and Miller, W. H.: Portasystemic shunts in 102 patients with portal hypertension. New Eng. J. Med., *274:*1290–1293, 1966.

Silen, W., Mawdsley, D. L., Weirich, W. L., and Harper, H. A.: Studies of hepatic function in dogs with Eck fistula or portacaval transposition. Arch. Surg., *74:*964–973, 1957.

Voorhees, A. B., Jr., Price, J. B., Jr., and Britton, R. C.: Portasystemic shunting procedures for portal hypertension. Twenty-six year experience in adults with cirrhosis of the liver. Amer. J. Surg., *119:*501–505, 1970.

Walker, R. M., Shaldon, C., and Vowles, K. D. J.: Late results of portacaval anastomosis. Lancet, *2:*727–730, 1961.

Wantz, G. E., and Payne, M. A.: Experience with portacaval shunt for portal hypertension. New Eng. J. Med., *265:*721–728, 1961.

Welch, C. S., and Ramos, A. G.: Results of portacaval shunts in the treatment of portal hypertension. Surgery, *41:*756–768, 1957.

Whipple, A. O.: The problem of portal hypertension in relation to the hepatosplenopathies. Ann. Surg., *122:*449–475, 1945.

Zuidema, G. D., and Child, C. G., III: Current status of portal decompression. Progr. Liver Dis. *1:*315–328, 1961.

postshunt encephalopathy

Brown, H.: Hepatic Failure. Springfield, Ill.: Charles C Thomas, 1970, 137 pp.

Brown, H., Trey, C., and McDermott, W. V., Jr.: Encephalopathy after portacaval shunting managed with lactulose. Amer. J. Surg., *119:*132–137, 1970.

Brown, H., Trey, C., and McDermott, W. V., Jr.: Lactulose treatment of hepatic encephalopathy in outpatients. Arch. Surg., *102:*25–27, 1971.

Kline, D. G., Crook, J. N., and Nance, F. C.: Eck fistula encephalography: Long-term studies in primates. Ann. Surg., *173:*97–103, 1971.

McDermott, W. V., Jr.: Metabolism and toxicity of ammonia. New Eng. J. Med., *257:*1076–1081, 1957.

McDermott, W. V., Jr., Barnes, B. A., Nardi, G. L., and Ackroyd, F. W.: Postshunt encephalopathy. Surg. Gynec. Obstet., *126:*585–590, 1968.

Nance, F. C., and Kline, D. G.: Eck's fistula encephalopathy in germfree dogs. Ann. Surg., *174:*856–862, 1971.

Price, J. B., Jr., Sawada, M., and Voorhees, A. B., Jr.: Clinical significance of intraluminal pH in intestinal ammonia transport. Amer. J. Surg., *119:*595–598, 1970.

Price, J. B., Jr., et al.: Determinants of ammonia tolerance in animals with and without portal systemic shunting. Surgery, *60:*701–709, 1966.

Price, J. B., Jr.: Effects of portal systemic shunting on intestinal absorption in the dog and in man. Surg. Gynec. Obstet., *125:*305–310, 1967.

Price, J. B., Jr., et al.: Mechanism and clinical significance of intestinal ammonia transport. Surg. Forum, *18:*331–333, 1967.

Resnick, R. H., et al.: A controlled trial of colon bypass in chronic hepatic encephalopathy. Gastroenterology, *54:*1057–1069, 1968.

Trey, C.: The critically ill child: Acute hepatic failure. Pediatrics, *45:*93–98, 1970.

Voorhees, A. B., Jr., and Price, J. B., Jr.: Surgical treatment of hepatic encephalopathy. Ann. N.Y. Acad. Sci., *170:*259–266, 1970.

Walshe, J. M.: Hepatic coma. Postgrad. Med. J., *32:*467–472, 1956.

Zuidema, G. D., et al.: Blood ammonia studies in monkeys before and after portacaval anastomosis. Arch. Surg., *85:*152–157, 1962.

postshunt peptic ulcer and gastric secretion

Anton, A. H., and Woodward, E. R.: High levels of blood histamine and peptic ulcer. In patient with portacaval shunt. Arch. Surg., *92:*96–97, 1966.

Castaneda, A., et al.: Antral hyperfunction following portacaval shunt. Surg. Forum, *11:*349–351, 1960.

Clarke, J. S.: Influence of the liver upon gastric secretion. Amer. J. Med., *29:*740–747, 1960.

Clarke, J. S., Hoffs, M., and El Farra, S.: The effect of portacaval transposition on Heidenhain pouch secretion in response to various stimuli. Surg. Forum, *10:*134–138, 1959.

Clarke, J. S., McKissock, P. K., and Cruze, K.: Studies on the site of origin of the agent causing hypersecretion in dogs with portacaval shunt. Surgery, *46:*48–55, 1959.

Clarke, J. S., et al.: Peptic ulcer following portacaval shunt. Ann. Surg., *148:*551-566, 1958.

Dubuque, T. J., Jr., Mulligan, L. V., and Neville, E. C.: Gastric secretion and peptic ulceration in the dog with portal obstruction and portacaval anastomosis. Surg. Forum, *8:*208-211, 1958.

Eiseman, B.: Histamine metabolism and liver disease. Amer. J. Dig. Dis., *7:*1099-1104, 1962.

Gerez, L., und Weiss, A.: Über die Magensaftsekretion bei Eckscher Fistel. Z. Ges. Exp. Med., *100:*281-288, 1937.

Gregory, R. A.: Gastric secretory responses after portal venous ligation. J. Physiol., *144:*123-137, 1958.

Hayaski, K., Rheault, M. J., Semb, L. S., and Nyhus, L. M.: The effect of splenocaval shunt on gastric secretion and liver function as compared with other shunting procedures in the dog. Surgery, *64:*1084-1091, 1968.

Irvine, W. T.: The liver, gastric secretion and histamine. Gastroenterology, *42:*337-339, 1962.

Irvine, W. T., Duthie, H. L., Ritchie, H. D., and Waton, N. G.: The liver's role in histamine absorption from the alimentary tract. Its possible importance in cirrhosis. Lancet, *1:*1064-1068, 1959.

Lebedinskaja, S. I.: Über die Magensekretion bei Eckschen Fistelhunden. Z. Ges. Exp. Med., *88:*264-270, 1933.

Liebowitz, H. R.: Peptic ulcer following portacaval shunt. Amer. J. Dig. Dis., *9:*605-617, 1964.

MacPherson, W. A., et al.: The importance of the antrum in gastric hypersecretion after shunt. Surg. Forum, *13:*271-273, 1962.

Orloff, M. J., and Windsor, C. W. O.: Effect of portacaval shunt on gastric acid secretion in dogs with liver disease, portal hypertension and massive ascites. Ann. Surg., *164:*69-80, 1966.

Peloso, O. A., Jacobson, S., and Silen, W.: Effect of changes in gastric secretion on protein tolerance after portacaval shunt. Amer. J. Surg., *112:*279-286, 1966.

Silen, W., and Eiseman, B.: The nature and cause of gastric hypersecretion following portacaval shunts. Surgery, *46:*38-47, 1959.

Silen, W., and Eiseman, B.: Evidence for histamine as the agent responsible for gastric hypersecretion after portacaval shunt. Surgery, *50:*213-219, 1961.

Silen, W., Hein, M. F., Albo, R. J., and Harper, H. A.: Influence of liver upon canine gastric secretion. Surgery, *54:*29-36, 1963.

Tabaqchali, S., and Dawson, A. M.: Peptic ulcer and gastric secretion in patients with liver disease. Gut, *5:*417-421, 1964.

Thompson, J. C.: Peptic ulcer associated with cirrhosis and portacaval shunt. *In* Orloff, M. J., et al.: The complications of cirrhosis of the liver. Ann. Int. Med., *66:*165-198 (189-192), 1967.

Thompson, J. C.: Alterations in gastric secretion after portacaval shunting. Amer. J. Surg., *117:*854-865, 1969.

Techniques of Shunting Procedures

CHAPTER 8

Although there are innumerable approaches and variations in the technique of constructing portal-systemic shunts, only one technique will be described in detail for each of the established shunting procedures since it would be nearly impossible and thoroughly confusing to interject segments of a number of different methods of achieving the same objective. Utilization by any surgeon of one particular technique, which he may well modify with growing experience, has the advantage of standardization and familiarity, both of which are important to a surgical team intent on performing a quick, effective and safe operative procedure.

The various types of shunts now in clinical usage are shown diagrammatically in Figure 7-1; selected point in the performance of the various procedures will also be utilized to amplify and clarify the verbal descriptions.

end-to-side portacaval shunt

The end-to-side portacaval shunt is certainly the most commonly used of the shunting procedures. Because of its relative simplicity and the effectiveness with which it will control bleeding from esophageal varices, it continues to be the operation of general utility.

The patient is positioned about 30 degrees off supine with a break just below the costal margin posteriorly. A long, lateral, subcostal incision is made, extending from the midline well out into the flank. This permits easy access to and exposure of the underside of the gastrohepatic ligament and to the infrahepatic vena cava. After the duodenum and hepatic flexure are mobilized the vena cava is identified by retroperitoneal dissection. In obese patients with ascites there is often a thick, edematous, fat layer retroperitoneally so that this maneuver is not always as simple as it sounds. By palpation of the right kidney, the aorta and vertebral column, the approximate location of the vena cava can be determined and the retroperitoneal opening placed accordingly. Because of the extensive spontaneous collateral circulation that develops in portal hypertension, there can be serious bleeding at this point in the operative procedure. Rather than attempt to establish meticulous hemostasis with cautery or ligatures, the operator is urged to proceed rapidly to the vena cava, packing the edges of the retroperitoneum with dry gauze used both for retraction and temporary hemostasis. Once the vena cava is identified and the retroperitoneum opened longitudinally, a whipping stitch of chromic catgut can be carried down both leaves of the retroperitoneum and some of the fatty tissue can be included behind it. This provides rapid, adequate and satisfactory hemostasis, which might literally take hours if attempts were made to identify individually and ligate or cauterize the multiple bleeding points (Fig. 8-1A).

Once this maneuver is completed, attention is directed to the underside of the gastrohepatic ligament where the peritoneal covering is incised posteriorly. Once the portal vein is initially identified and appears patent by palpation, it is carefully dissected out from its bed behind the common bile duct and the hepatic artery. If preoperative arteriography has not been carried out, the surgeon will wish to ascertain that the hepatic artery lies in its normal position rather than assuming a relatively common anomalous course in which the right hepatic artery enters the liver behind the portal vein. Dissection of the portal vein is continued proximally and distally; this dissection is greatly facilitated by the maneuver shown in Figure 8-1B in which two poms held in Moynihan clamps are used to keep the gastrohepatic ligament on stretch and to retract the common bile duct from its position overlying the portal vein. Caution should be exercised relative to the location of the pyloric vein: It should be ligated carefully and divided if it appears in the course of the anatomic dissection; otherwise, extremely troublesome bleeding may occur since this vein retracts to an inaccessible position. Once satisfactory mobilization of the portal vein has been carried out from the bifurcation at the hilus of the liver to the point where the portal vein passes behind the pancreas, the surgeon can then determine how much further mobilization of the vena cava will be required.

The anatomic relationship of the portal vein to the vena cava is extremely variable and depends on the distortion that has occurred from the process of regeneration in the cirrhotic liver. Frequently, the caudate lobe hypertrophies and presents a barrier between the vena cava and the portal vein; also, the angle at which the portal vein enters the liver relative to the course of the vena cava behind the liver varies considerably. Sometimes they may run nearly parallel courses, but on other occasions they may be almost at right angles to one another.

Further mobilization of the vena cava is then carried out, if necessary, to construct a portacaval shunt without tension; this may necessitate ligation of the lower one or two small hepatic veins and occasionally a wedge resection of a portion of intervening caudate lobe (Fig. 8-1A). While it is important to clean the vena cava by sharp dissection, too vigorous and meticulous an approach to this will leave the cava without a very tough adventitial covering, which of course makes it much more likely to tear during the construction of the anastomosis.

At this point, splanchnic and hepatic pressure measurements can be taken, not only for general informational purposes, but to use as partial determinants of the type of shunt to be constructed. A medium Blalock clamp is then placed across the portal vein as it disappears behind the pancreas in such a way that it does not angulate the portal vein. Next a heavy ligature is placed as high as possible around the hepatic end of the portal vein and a right angle clamp applied proximal to this. The portal vein is then divided with sharp scissors and a suture ligature fixed around the right angle clamp before it is removed.

At this point a Satinsky clamp is placed at an appropriate position on the anterior medial aspect of the vena cava, the exact location to be determined by the angle at which the portal vein may be swung down to meet it. Since one of the real disasters of the operation may occur if the Satinsky clamp slips, it is advisable to place two holding ligatures as indicated in Figure 8-1C and to tie heavy tape around the middle of the clamp so that it cannot be sprung inadvertently during construction of the shunt.

The size of the ellipse of the wall of the vena cava which is then to be removed for construction of the shunt remains a controversial subject. The high incidence of encephalopathy would indicate that as large a shunt as possible should not be constructed; on the other hand, one must be sure to achieve adequate decompression since the primary objective of the operation is to prevent further bleeding from esophageal varices. In our opinion, the shunt should measure approximately 1.5 cm. in diameter, so an appropriate ellipse of cava is then removed with a Potts scissors, and 5-0 Mersilene is used to construct the anastomosis. A holding suture is placed through the superior end of the two vessels and an everting, continuous mattress suture carried out from above down (Fig. 8-1D). When the lower end of the projected anastomosis has been reached, another holding stitch is applied at the lower junction, and both these holding stitches are tied down securely. By gentle traction on the posterior suture line the continuous suture can be snugged up and an everting approximation of the intima of the portal vein and vena cava accomplished. The two ends of the posterior row are then tied.

An anterior row is now begun from above down, using the same technique of everting mattress stitch, which is, of course, a great deal easier in the anterior than the posterior row. Rather than continuing the anterior stitch throughout the entire length of the anterior portion of the anastomosis, it is interrupted at a midpoint and another continuous everting suture started from below. When these are in proximity, the Blalock clamps should be released temporarily to flush out any

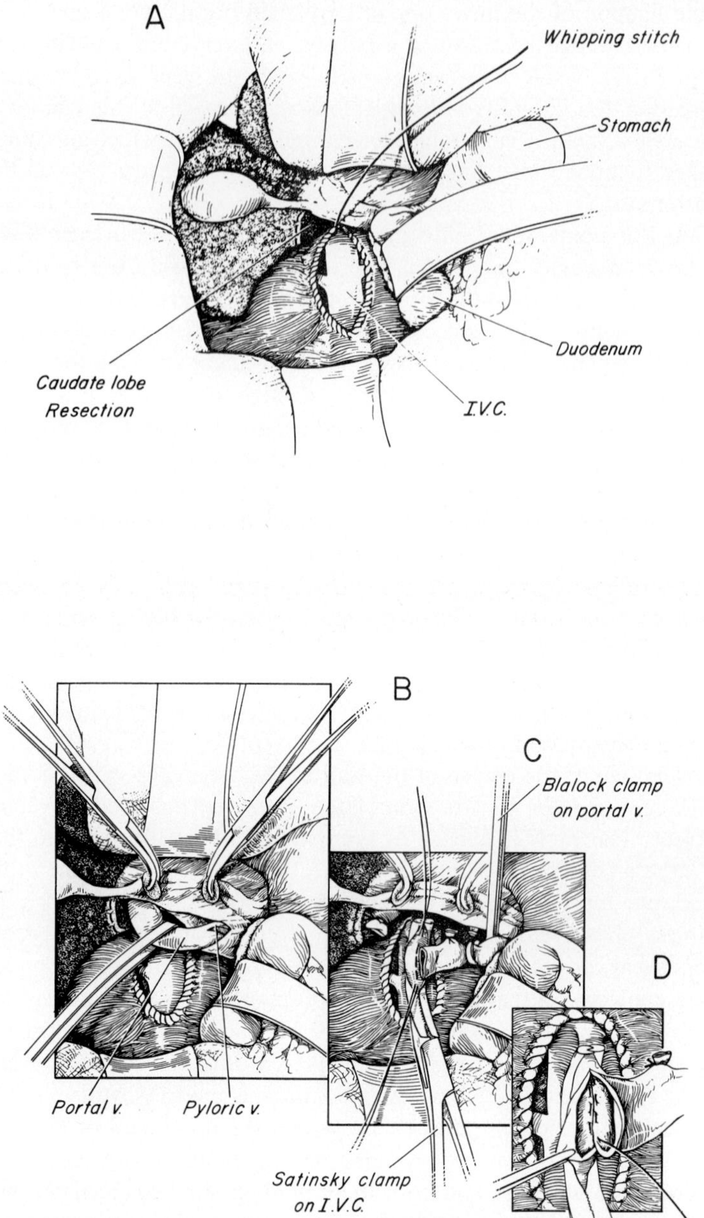

FIG. 8-1. Techniques of shunt operations: A, Exposing the inferior vena cava. B, Exposing the portal vein. C and D, End-to-side anastomosis. E, Side-to-side shunt using the Kimoto triple-bladed clamp. F, Double portacaval shunt with division of pancreas. G, Splenorenal shunt

E

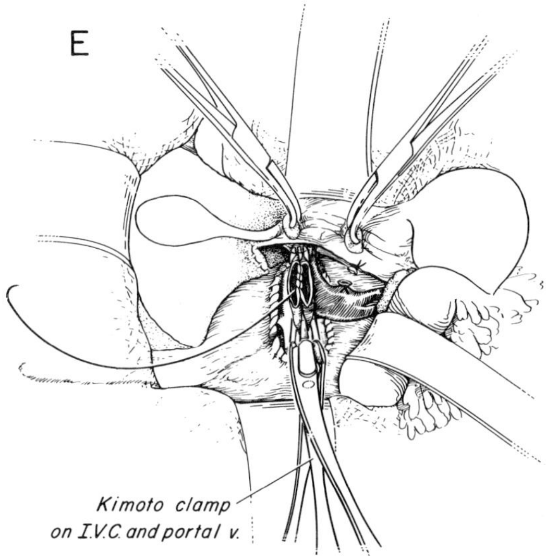
Kimoto clamp
on I.V.C. and portal v.

F

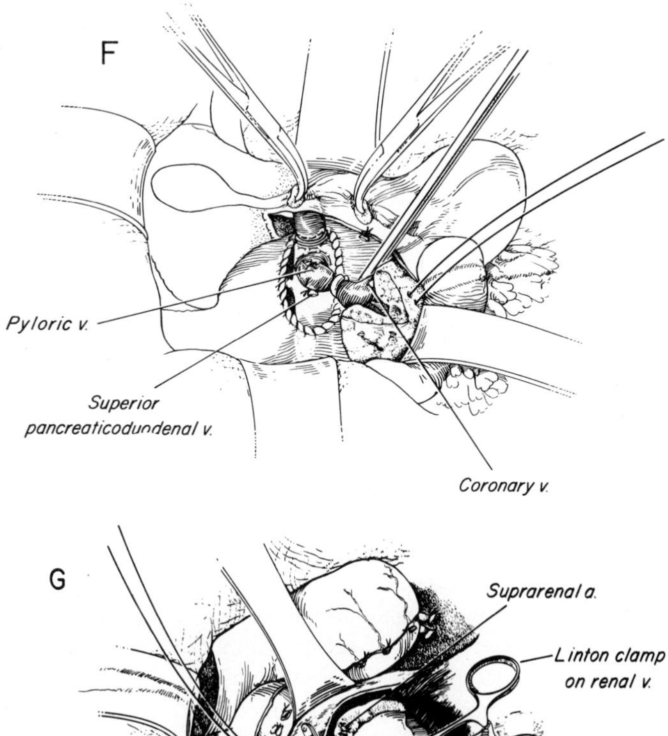
Pyloric v.
Superior
pancreaticoduodenal v.
Coronary v.

G

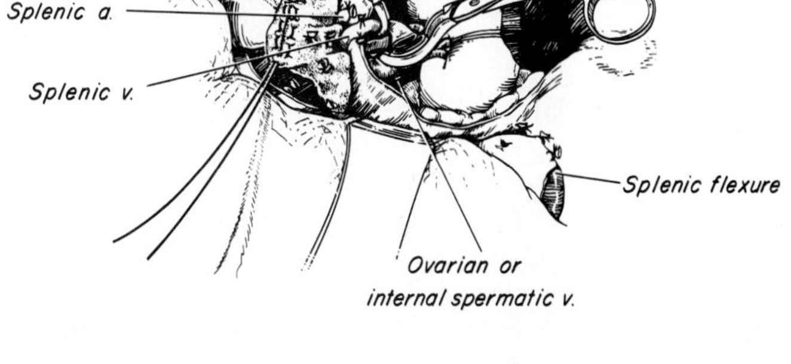
Suprarenal a.
Linton clamp
on renal v.
Splenic a.
Splenic v.
Splenic flexure
Ovarian or
internal spermatic v.

clot that may have formed in the portal vein and to determine that a free flow does exist. The anterior row is then snugged up and tied, the Blalock clamp removed and the suture lined checked for bleeding points; finally, the Satinsky clamp is removed and the operation is completed.

Various types of closure of the abdominal incision may be used, but in our hands, closely spaced, heavy nylon sutures through all layers of the abdominal wall supplemented by continuous catgut closure of the various peritoneal and fascial layers are the safest in these frequently debilitated and malnourished patients.

side-to-side portacaval shunt

The incision and preliminary dissection described for the end-to-side portacaval shunt are certainly applicable to the next two operative procedures and need not be repeated. Once dissection of the vena cava and portal vein has been completed, a decision must be made whether a side-to-side or double portacaval shunt should or could be constructed. Both achieve the same physiologic end results, although slightly greater decompression of both the intrahepatic and the splanchnic bed can be accomplished by a double end-to-side portacaval shunt. If the distance between the two veins is not great, the anastomosis can be constructed without a high degree of tension.

When the vena cava is completely mobilized from its bed, a side-to-side shunt is the simplest from a technical point of view. It is frequently necessary in both side-to-side and double end-to-side portacaval shunts to resect a wedge of caudate lobe as shown in Figure 8-1A. The Kimoto triple-bladed clamp is very useful in constructing a side-to-side shunt if sufficient cuff of vena cava and portal vein can be drawn up into the two sections of the clamp (Fig. 8-1E). If tension is too great and this is not possible, or if slipping of the cuff occurs in the clamp, it is better to use two Blalock clamps on the portal vein and a Satinsky clamp on the vena cava. Once the two vessels are approximated and opened over a distance of about 2 cm., an anastomosis is constructed similar to that described for the end-to-side portacaval shunt except that a running suture is ordinarily used on the posterior wall because of its greater simplicity under the circumstances; although the everting mattress suture is theoretically more desirable, no difference in terms of thrombosis of the shunt has been noted with use of a simple running suture.

double end-to-side shunt

Technically, this shunt is used if there is a long segment of portal vein available and considerable distance and angulation in the anatomic positions of the portal vein and vena cava. It is almost invariably necessary to resect a portion of the enlarged caudate lobe, and often division of the pancreas (as shown in Fig. 8-1F) may be required to obtain an adequate length of portal vein. The divided edges of the pancreas are closed with mattress sutures of catgut (in cases in which this has been done, no complications relative to this maneuver have been noted to date), but great care should be taken not to tear the pancreaticoduodenal veins entering the portal vein behind the pancreas. Anastomosis of the hepatic side of the divided portal vein and the anterior wall of the vena cava is usually carried out first; the second anastomosis of the splanchnic side of the portal vein is placed more medially and inferiorly as shown in Figure 8-1F. The details of the anastomosis itself are similar to that already described.

splenorenal shunt

Exposure for the construction of a splenorenal shunt is achieved by a thoracoabdominal incision extending from the midline across the chest wall in the line of the 10th or 11th rib, whichever appears from the configuration of the rib flare to give appropriate exposure of the area of the hilus of the spleen. The diaphragm is incised in the line of the incision. After appropriate exploration, the spleen is mobilized by dividing the lienocolic, lienophrenic and lienogastric ligaments, all of which usually contain enlarged veins under increased portal pressure. The retroperitoneal attachments of the spleen are also quite vascular and when incised in order to enter the retroperitoneal area behind the spleen will bleed vigorously. Rather than attempt individual ligations in this area, it is much more satisfactory to achieve hemostasis with a whipping stitch of chromic catgut extending from the diaphragm to the splenic flexure.

As the spleen is mobilized and the lesser omentum entered after the lower vasa brevia is divided, the splenic artery can be identified. After pressure measurements have been taken in the splenic pulp, the splenic artery is clamped, cut and doubly ligated. Dissection of the splenic vein can be carried out at the point where the venous tributaries of the spleen have collected into a common trunk; in portal hypertension, this vein is usually dilated and very thin walled and may be injured easily. It is therefore preferable although somewhat more tedious to dissect out the two main branches of the splenic vein, remove the spleen and then begin dissection towards the main splenic vein along one of the bifurcations. The splenic vein branches can be used for traction with holding ligatures during dissection. Most of the tributaries entering the main splenic vein emanate from a groove in the pancreas in which the splenic vein lies posteriorly. This portion of dissection should not be hurried; the individual branches should be isolated, ligated and cut with care since damage to the splenic vein wall at this point may not only be irreparable but also may destroy the opportunity for a satisfactory shunt.

Once an adequate segment of splenic vein has been isolated, attention is next directed to the hilus of the kidney where the renal veins and renal artery can be identified by dissection in the perirenal fat. Anomalies of the renal circulation are relatively common; except for bifid vessels, the only one that is pertinent to this operation is the passage of an inferior renal artery branch to the lower pole of the kidney crossing the renal vein and interfering with the positioning of the anastomosis. This inferior pole branch may be ligated and divided to achieve adequate access to the splenic vein; the occasional renal infarct that results seems to cause no serious damage. In order to obtain satisfactory mobilization of the renal vein, it is usually necessary to divide the spermatic (or ovarian) vein as it enters from below. A smaller adrenal vein entering superiorly should also be ligated to achieve a free and mobile renal vein for construction of the shunt.

Once the renal vein is mobilized, one can ascertain whether a sufficient length of splenic vein has been dissected free to swing down to the renal vein in a gently curving arc without tension. Because of anatomic variations it is sometimes necessary to resect a portion of the tail of the pancreas in such a way that a fish-mouth incision permits easy closure of the transected tail of the pancreas. A bulldog clamp is placed across the splenic vein and the ligated end cut with a Potts scissors at an angle that permits it to lie easily against the anterosuperior surface of the renal vein. A segment of the anterior wall of the renal vein is then drawn up into a partially occluded clamp designed by Linton (Fig. 8-1G) or a small Kimoto clamp and an ellipse excised sufficient to match the transected end of the splenic vein. Anastomosis is carried out with an everting, continuous, mattress suture in a fashion similar to that described for the anastomosis of the end of the portal vein to the vena cava. After liver biopsy and postoperative measurements of splenic vein pressure, the abdomen and chest are closed in the usual fashion as described previously. The chest cavity is drained through the 10th or 11th interspace; drainage of the left subphrenic area is not carried out unless the tail of the pancreas has been resected.

mesocaval shunt

Through either a transverse or a right paramedian incision the superior mesenteric vein is identified at the ligament of Treitz and carefully dissected upward behind the transverse mesocolon, retractors being used to elevate the transverse colon and its attachments (Fig. 8-2A). This dissection is the key to a successful procedure, and in portal hypertension the vein is, as the splenic vein, distended and thin walled. Ordinarily the superior mesenteric vein is sufficiently long for a satisfactory anastomosis, but occasionally one will find a vein either thrombosed or dividing into multiple branches shortly after its emergence from behind the pancreas so that satisfactory anastomosis is not possible. If the superior mesenteric vein is suitable for a shunt, attention is directed towards dissecting the vena cava either

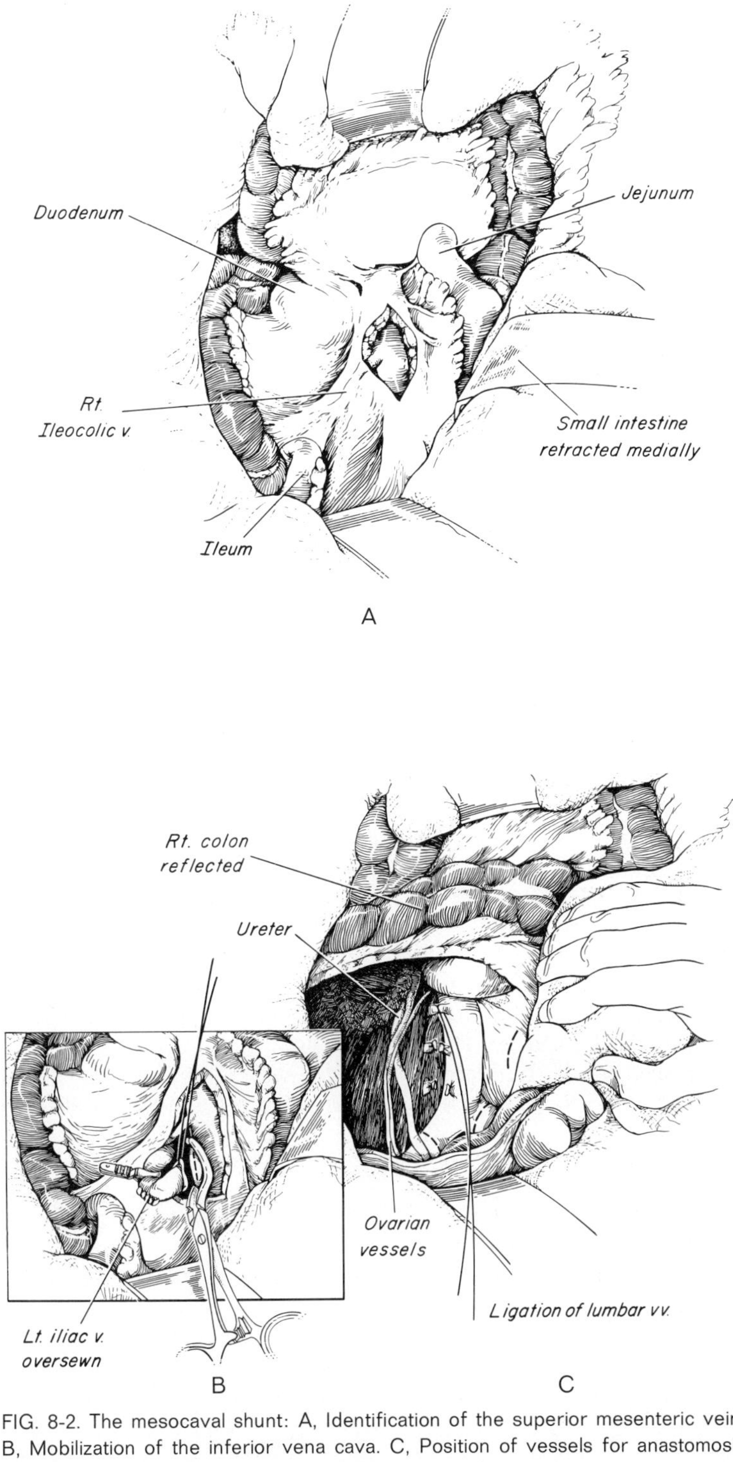

FIG. 8-2. The mesocaval shunt: A, Identification of the superior mesenteric vein. B, Mobilization of the inferior vena cava. C, Position of vessels for anastomosis

by mobilizing the right colon towards the midline or by proceeding directly through the retroperitoneum to the left of the superior mesenteric vein. The vena cava and the two common iliac veins are then dissected free, and lumbar branches are ligated as they are encountered (Fig. 8-2B). The left common iliac vein is transected and oversewn at its junction with the inferior vena cava. The right common iliac vein is dissected for a few centimeters before transection and ligation to give more adequate length to the entire venous segment. The end of the right common iliac vein with the vena cava can be drawn through a hole in the mesocolon towards the superior mesenteric vein and an end-to-side anastomosis carried out with instruments similar to those described for the splenorenal shunt (Fig. 8-2C). Recently, Drapanas described a series of successful mesocaval shunts in which a Dacron graft was used to provide a conduit between the vessels. Apparently patency has been maintained, and, since the veins remain in continuity, the operative procedure is considerably simplified.

renoportal shunt

If the distance or the angle between the portal vein and the inferior vena cava precludes a satisfactory approximation, the left renal vein can be dissected for a sufficient length and then divided for an end-to-side anastomosis to the portal vein. This functions as a side-to-side shunt, and no problems relative to renal function have arisen secondary to ligation of the vein at this distance from the kidney.

bibliography

Child, C. G., III: The Liver and Portal Hypertension. Philadelphia, W. B. Saunders Co., 1964, 231 pp.

Davidson, C. S.: Liver Pathophysiology. Its Relevance to Human Disease. Boston, Little, Brown and Company, 1970, 279 pp.

Madding, G. F., and Kennedy, P. A.: Trauma to the Liver. 2nd Ed. Philadelphia, W. B. Saunders Co., 1971, 186 pp.

McDermott, W. V., Jr.: Bleeding esophageal varices. *In* Conn, H. F. (Ed.): Current Therapy. Philadelphia, W. B. Saunders Co., 1968, pp. 287–288.

Nardi, G. L., and Zuidema, G. D. (Eds.): Surgery. A Concise Guide to Clinical Practice. 3rd Ed. Boston, Little, Brown and Company, 1972, 1155 pp.

Schwartz, S. E.: Surgical Diseases of the Liver. New York, McGraw-Hill Book Company, 1964, 387 pp.

Sedgwick, C. E., and Poulantzas, J. K.: Portal Hypertension. Boston, Little, Brown and Company, 1967, 257 pp.

Tumors of the Liver and Hepatic Resection

CHAPTER 9

There are many benign and malignant tumors of the liver; their classification is given in Table 9-1. Many of these are of academic interest; no attempt will be made in this section to discuss specific pathologic characteristics of each since this information is easily available in a number of standard texts and articles to which reference has been made in the bibliography. Rather, an effort will be made to concentrate on the particular clinical characteristics of those tumors that are most likely to come to the attention of the surgeon. At this point, however, it is important to note that a number of nodules of differing types occur in the liver, the only real significance of which is the distinct possibility that they can be mistaken for metastatic disease; therefore, an unnecessarily gloomy prognosis can be given to a patient who has had a successful resection within the gastrointestinal tract. Mixter and Mixter emphasized this point some years ago and pointed out that small hemangiomas, bile duct proliferations, calcified cysts, tumors, fibromas and many other innocuous lesions may lead the surgeon to a false impression and prognosis. Thus, a microscopic diagnosis is mandatory.

benign tumors

Among the benign tumors of the liver that may present indications for major hepatic resection, a *cavernous hemangioma* is perhaps the most frequent. While multiple, small capillary hemangiomas are quite frequently found and are of no particular significance, these large, vascular hemangiomas may reach unusual size and present a very real hazard to the patient's life. The extraordinary vascularity of these lesions is such that a number of reports exist on patients who bled

TABLE 9-1. Classification of Tumors of the Liver*

A. Benign
   1. Parenchymal (hepatoadenomas, cholangioadenomas, mixed tumors)
   2. Mesodermal (capillary angioma, cavernous hemangioma, lymphangioma, endothelioma)
   3. Cysts
      a. Congenital (solitary, diffuse)
      b. Parasitic (Echinococcus)
      c. Neoplastic (cystadenomas, dermoids)
   4. Miscellaneous (teratoma, hamartoma, fibromas, lipomas, adrenal cell rests)
B. Malignant
   1. Primary (hepatocarcinoma, cholangiocarcinoma)
   2. Metastatic (adenocarcinoma, carcinoid, insulinoma, etc.)

*Modified from Edmondson and from Manson et al.

to death after an open biopsy and inability to control the subsequent bleeding. Trauma may rupture the tumor and cause fatal hemorrhage. Many of these lesions will result in severe thrombocytopenia because of the action on circulating platelets, and this leads to a secondary problem in addition to the primary threat of traumatic rupture. Repeated infarctions within the tumor may occur with attacks of unexplained pain. In our own experience, a large, cavernous hemangioma in the dome of the right lobe of the liver was the source of recurrent bouts of fever of unknown origin apparently associated with successive episodes of infarction. Therefore, very justifiable indications exist for a radical surgical approach to these particular tumors despite their biologically innocuous nature. If the cavernous hemangioma proves inoperable because of its anatomic location or the condition of the patient, x-ray therapy may be used. Occasionally this has resulted in decrease of the tumor mass.

Hamartoma of the liver is an interesting lesion, controversial in terms of nomenclature and categorization as a true neoplastic lesion. Nonetheless, it reaches enormous size and presents serious problems relative to the displacement of abdominal viscera. One occasionally encounters unusual features associated with hamartoma of the liver. Significant polycythemia, corrected by removal of the tumor, has been described, and, therefore, this tumor can probably be grouped with others known to secrete an erythropoietic substance. With an unusually large hamartoma in our own series (Fig. 9-1), a serum albumin level of 6.0 gm. per 100 ml. was an unusual preoperative feature and suggested that the multiple nodular hyperplasia of this particular tumor was extremely active in the synthesis of serum albumin.

Of the cystic tumors of the liver that may require surgical intervention, the *echinococcus cyst* is particularly common in many parts

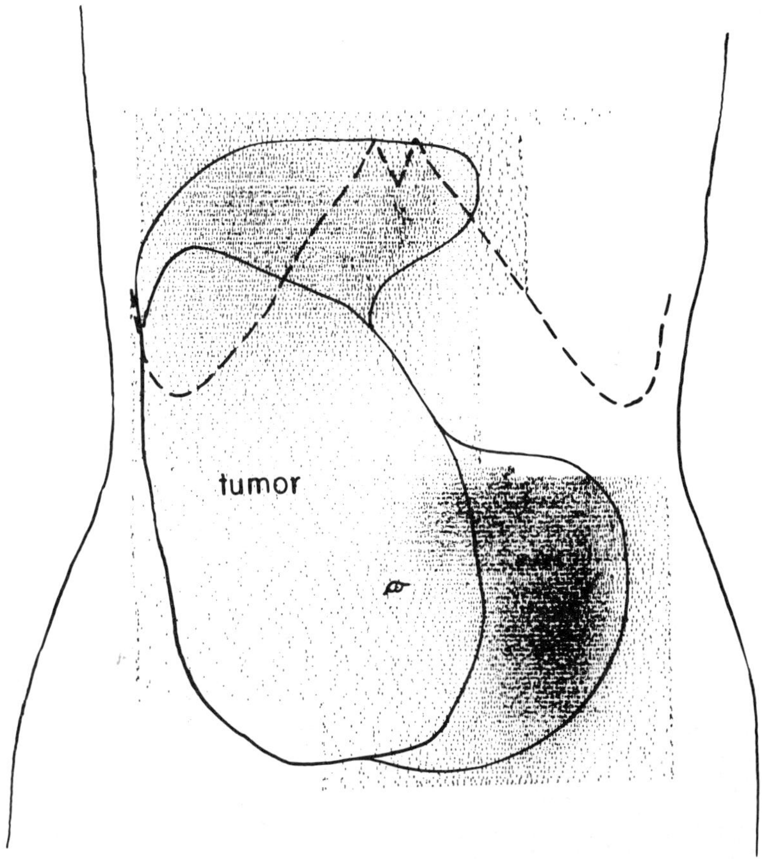

FIG. 9-1. Scintiscan of large hamartoma of the liver

of the world such as Greece, Argentina and Australia. In the continental United States this lesion is usually found only in people who have had exposure in areas of the world in which the Echinococcus is endemic, but obviously the parasite does exist within this country since cases have been reported in individuals who had never left these shores. Detailed literature on the life cycle of this parasite is easily available, and for purposes of this text, reference will be made only to some of the details important to the surgeon facing this particular tumor. If the cyst is located in an area easily accessible to wide resection, this procedure is probably preferable in a good risk patient. If, however, the cyst overlaps the normal anatomic divisions of the liver, there are other approaches such as aspiration, drainage or marsupialization. One of the risks of aspiration and drainage of these tumors is the contamination of the peritoneal cavity with active parasites, but this can be controlled by careful instillation of 10 per cent formaldehyde to kill the parasites before further approach is made to the tumor. Once the active spores have been killed or if the cyst has been rendered inactive by previous bacterial infection, as indicated by the purulent nature of the contents, then the cyst may be opened, the lining stripped away and the cyst cavity either obliterated by suturing or exteriorized by marsupialization. Regardless of the viability of the spores, the danger of anaphylactic reaction is such that precautions should always be taken to avoid spillage of the cyst contents into the free peritoneal cavity.

malignant tumors

Of the malignant tumors of the liver, *metastatic carcinoma* is by far the most common encountered by the surgeon. While the liver is the favorite site for seeding of tumors from a variety of primary sources, it is relatively unusual to find a case in which an apparently solitary metastasis has occurred that might be considered for resection (Fig. 9-2). Ordinarily, this situation will arise only in association with tumors originating in the colon, and resection should be considered only in instances in which the nature of the primary cancer itself would offer a reasonably favorable prognosis. Even then, the results

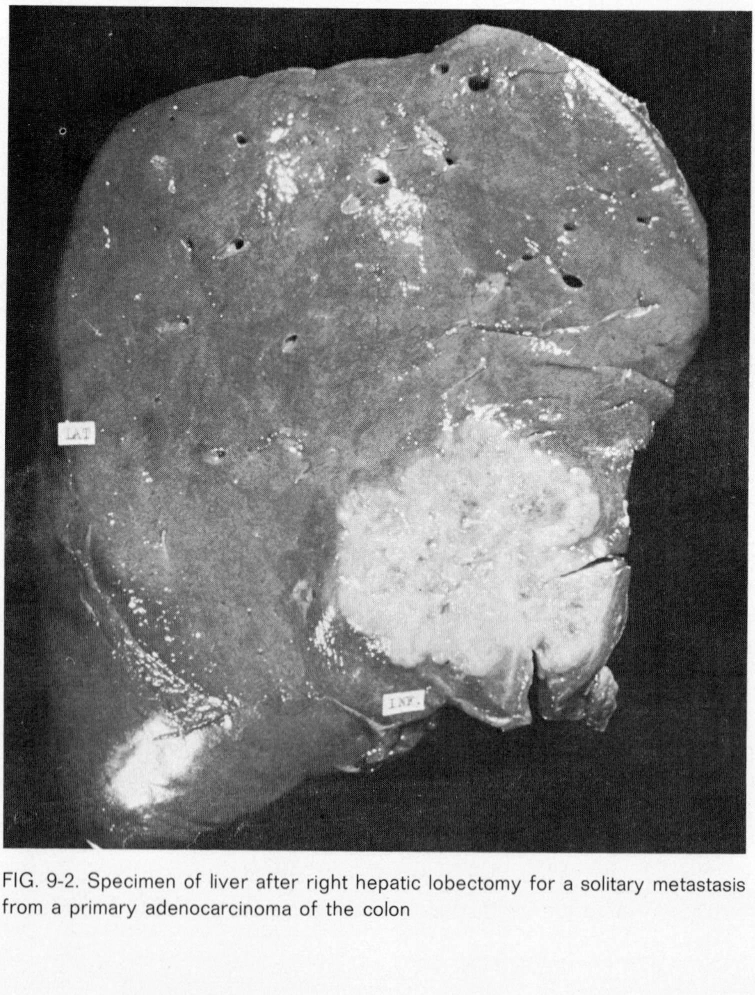

FIG. 9-2. Specimen of liver after right hepatic lobectomy for a solitary metastasis from a primary adenocarcinoma of the colon

nave not been impressive in terms of total cures after resection of apparently solitary secondary lesions, but no reported series is large enough yet to define with exactitude the chances of eradicating this type of metastatic disease. It would appear, however, that in carefully selected cases a major hepatic resection may be indicated, and long term survivals have already been reported. In 1961, Brasfield reported the first five year survival, and several additional cases have since reached this standard landmark of cancer survival.

Although not as common, the primary malignant tumors of the liver (hepatocarcinoma or cholangiocarcinoma) are of particular interest and, if resectable, may well be cured by wide excision. The hepatocarcinoma, commonly referred to as a *hepatoma,* has aroused widespread interest because of the number of studies now available suggesting various exciting possibilities in terms of carcinogenesis. In the United States, hepatoma occurring in the normal liver is ordinarily found in the young adult, and early metastasis is not frequent so that a reasonable chance of cure may be expected from radical resection. In association with cirrhosis, however, the disease is usually multicentric in nature and ordinarily presents as a terminal event in the course of a longstanding cirrhotic process. This type of malignant disease is more common in hemochromatosis and in cryptogenic cirrhosis, particularly of the postnecrotic variety, than it is in the nutritional or alcoholic cirrhosis.

Most of the observations related to carcinogenic factors in hepatoma have come from animal studies or from observations made on the continent of Africa where hepatoma ranks very high in incidence among all the malignant disease encountered (Fig. 9-3). A series of articles edited by Burdette will serve as an excellent review in depth of this fascinating problem and will provide an extensive bibliography for further study of the various exciting leads concerned with hepatic oncogenesis. Demographic observations in Africa by Alpert and his associates from the Boston City Hospital would indicate that the prevalence of the disease is caused by environmental rather than genetic factors (Fig. 9-4). In areas in which grain and ground nuts form a staple part of the African diet and are stored for long periods, hepatoma and cirrhosis are both frequent in the population. It has been shown that *Aspergillus flavus,* known to be a contaminant of these staples, contains aflatoxins that produce hepatic carcinoma in the rainbow trout and in many species of experimental animals. The cycad nut and the germinal center of the palm have also been shown to have potential for experimental production of hepatic carcinoma. These provocative observations are being actively and vigorously pursued in a number of areas. A cancer research unit supported by the National Cancer Institute and located in Uganda has described the very high incidence of the AU antigen and of alpha-fetoprotein in patients with hepatoma.

Alpha-fetoprotein (AFP) is formed by embryonal liver cells but disappears after birth and is not detectable in normal adults. AFP has been detected when there is postresection hepatic regeneration

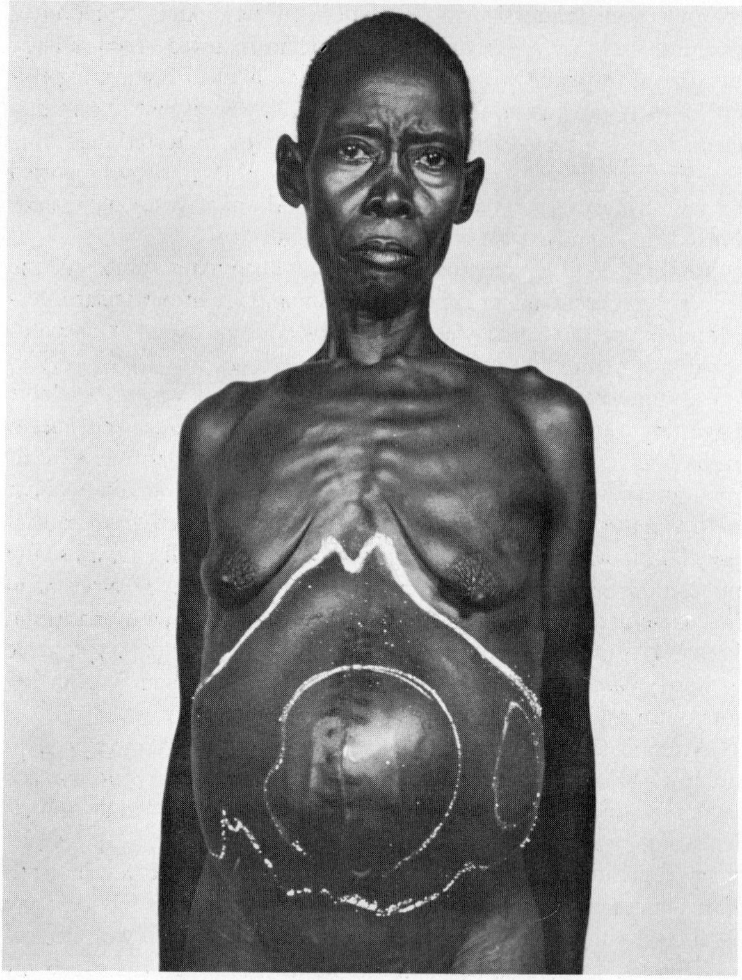

FIG. 9-3. Typical case of primary hepatoma in Uganda

in the experimental animal. Otherwise, AFP appeared to be almost specific for primary hepatomas and is found in the sera of the majority of patients with this malignant tumor. Ordinarily, it is not found in metastatic cancer of the liver, but recently three cases of gastric carcinoma with liver metastases were reported as showing detectable amounts of AFP. The presumption was that since the liver is an outgrowth of the foregut, malignant neoplasms of the upper gastrointestinal tract might demonstrate the same capacity for the synthesis of AFP as does the malignant liver tumor. Embryonal gonadal tumors may also secrete AFP, and there are isolated reports of positive findings in association with hepatitis, cirrhosis, pancreatic carcinoma and liver metastases. In another recently described case in which there was demonstrable AFP the patient had both gastric carcinoma and prostatic cancer, raising, of course, the question which of the malignant conditions was the source of the abnormal protein. Despite the lack of absolute specificity of AFP for primary hepatoma, it is only rarely found in other malignant growths and in other conditions, and the great majority of patients who demonstrate this fetal protein have undifferentiated malignant hepatocytes; therefore, it is valuable in screening tests in this particular clinical situation.

Sixty-eight per cent of patients with proven hepatocellular carcinoma had demonstrable levels of alpha-fetoprotein in their blood, and with increasing sensitivity of the test, this percentage will probably increase. (In one particularly interesting patient, a positive test reverted after resection of a large hepatoma only to become positive again a few months later as tumor recurred in the remaining left lobe.) In this same group of patients, 44 per cent had positive reactions to the hepatitis-associated antigen in contrast to 71 per cent of controls. Somewhat surprisingly, there was no significant difference between those patients with coexisting cirrhosis and those in whom the hepatoma developed in an otherwise normal liver.

With the amount of effort and interest focused on this particular tumor, it is inevitable that the coming months and years will produce intriguing information relative to the hepatoma and possibly applicable to carcinogenesis in a number of other malignant tumors. In addition to the great interest aroused by the demographic observa-

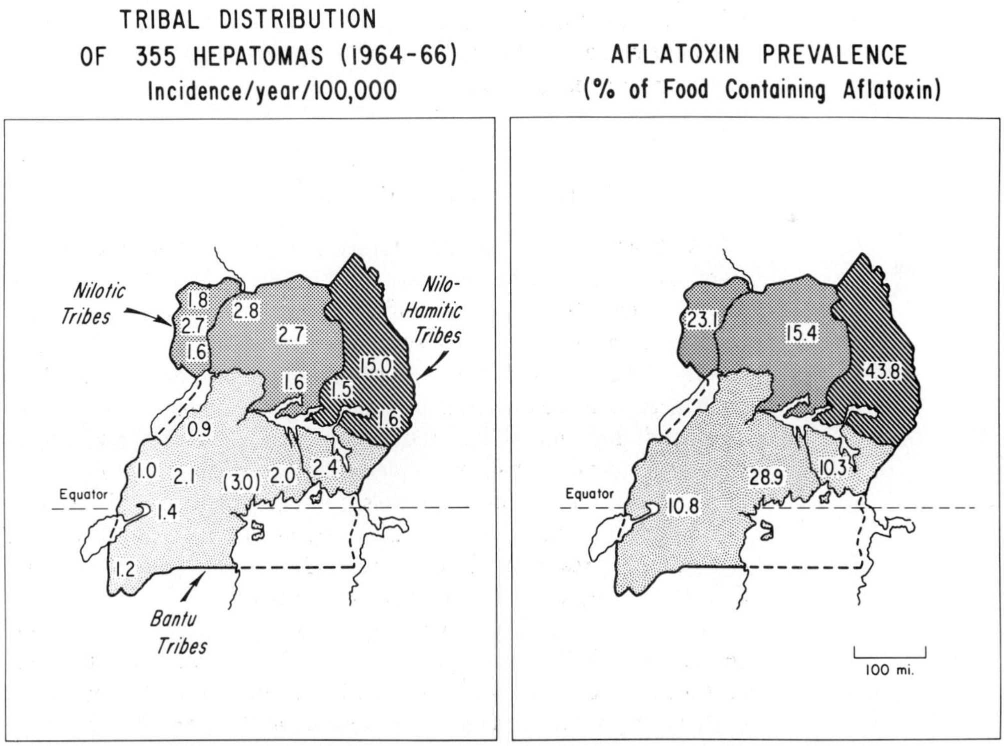

FIG. 9-4. Hepatoma in Uganda. (Reproduced from Alpert, M. S. R., et al.: Association between Aflatoxin Content of Food and Hepatoma Frequency in Uganda. Cancer *28*:253–260, 1971, with permission of the Publisher)

tions, the implications of carcinogenesis by mycotoxins and other substances associated with food intake and the peculiar relationship of hepatoma to nonalcoholic cirrhosis, this tumor has also been associated with bizarre endocrine abnormalities. Hypoglycemia is relatively common, and its occurrence is attributed to the peculiar avidity of large hepatomas for glucose in the synthesis of glycogen. Polycythemia is a well recognized phenomenon associated with some hepatomas. Hypercalcemia with evidence of increased parathyroid hormone-like polypeptide has been described, and evidence of the secretion of an insulin-like hormone has also been presented.

Carcinoma of the biliary tract is not ordinarily considered in the classification of primary hepatic tumors, and the scope of this particular text does not include a discussion of the extrahepatic biliary tree. Nonetheless, in terms of surgery of the liver and hepatic resection, it is important to note that tumors of the right or left hepatic duct may be amenable to major hepatic resection, and if the tumor can be encompassed with a reasonable margin, the prognosis should be good since these frequently are slow growing, relatively benign tumors.

Carcinoma of the gallbladder is ordinarily considered an incurable lesion because of the propensity for early metastasis both to nodes and within the right lobe of the liver, but five year survivals have already been reported following right hepatic lobectomy. Certainly all indications would be that this particular procedure offers the only real hope of cure of any but an occult, very early, incidentally removed carcinoma of the gallbladder wall.

results of treatment of liver cancer

With scattered notable exceptions, the treatment of cancer of the liver, either primary or metastatic, has not been very effective. Brasfield has recently reported six of 33 patients who had varying types of hepatic resection who have survived more than five years. Our own results (Table 9-2) are even less encouraging; of 15 patients in whom right hepatic lobectomy was carried out for malignant disease, only five are living and well at the present time, and only one has, as yet, survived more than five years. The occasional apparent "cure" in these and other reports indicates, however, that surgical resection is applicable in selected cases and certainly is the only chance for any effective treatment since neither radiation nor systemic chemotherapy has any role even in terms of palliation.

Regional infusion chemotherapy, however, may achieve some degree of palliation, although an adequately controlled and randomized study is not available for verification of some clinical impressions. Cady has reported on the technique, which in this procedure is particularly important, and has achieved a median patency time of 12 weeks with 18 of 73 patients maintaining patency for over six months. In this group of 73 patients with disseminated metastatic disease treated

TABLE 9-2. Results in 24 Cases of Elective Right Hepatic Lobectomy*

Indication	Metastatic Cancer 7	Cancer of Gallbladder 3	Hepatoma 5	Benign Tumor 6	Abscess or Cyst 3
Operative survival	6	2	5	6	2
Late deaths	4 Recurrent Disease 3 mos.–3 yrs.	2 Recurrent Disease 7 mos.–2 yrs.	2 Recurrent Disease 6 mos.–2 yrs.	0	1 Unrelated Causes 3 yrs.
Living and well	2 1–4 yrs.	0	3 6 mos.–6 yrs.	6 9 mos.–5 yrs.	1 2 yrs.

*Operative mortality—12%

by regional infusion with FUDR, the median survival time was over nine months as compared to an untreated group in Watkins' series whose median survival was four and one-half months; both objective and subjective improvement were described in a number of cases. In terms of complications, 11 patients developed some type of peptic ulceration, and migration of the catheter occurred in seven.

In summary, "cures" of primary or secondary hepatic cancer are possible but infrequent after surgical resection; some palliation may be achieved by regional perfusion, but radiation or systemic chemotherapy has little to offer.

techniques of hepatic resection

right hepatic lobectomy

The patient is placed in a position approximately 30 degrees from the supine so that easy access to the right side of the chest may be had by extension from an original abdominal incision. Through a right paramedian incision, abdominal exploration is carried out to determine the feasibility of the planned procedure. The incision can then be angled across the right chest wall, preferably over the fifth rib, entering the right lower cavity by removing the rib. If the thoracic component of the incision is much lower than this, access to the vena cava as it passes through the diaphragm and thus to the entrance of the major right and left hepatic veins may be difficult. The diaphragm is then divided in the line of the incision, thus exposing the vena cava and the liver, behind which it passes in its course through the right upper quadrant. Dissection of the gastrohepatic ligament is then carried out in such a way as to identify and isolate the hepatic artery, portal vein and common bile duct with their major branches.

Preliminary arteriography (Fig. 9-5) will be of tremendous help in prior recognition of the very frequent anomalies of the arterial supply to the liver. Since excellent descriptions of these anomalies are available in the anatomic treatise by Michels, it seems unnecessary to redescribe these in any detail. The most frequent anomaly (20 per cent) is the aberrant origin of the right hepatic artery from the superior mesenteric in such a way that it courses behind the portal vein and the common bile duct instead of being in its usual position medial to these structures. In this particular anomalous situation the left hepatic artery is very likely to arise from the left gastric and enter the liver separately.

Once identification of the anatomy of the gastrohepatic ligament has been achieved and identifying tapes passed around the right branches of the major structures, attention is directed to the lateral aspect of the liver where the peritoneum is divided, the retroperitoneal portion of the liver exposed and the right lobe retracted medially by the assistant. This maneuver will expose the retrohepatic vena cava

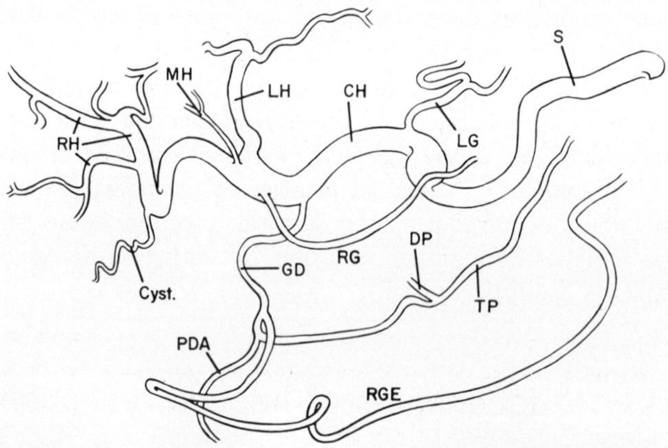

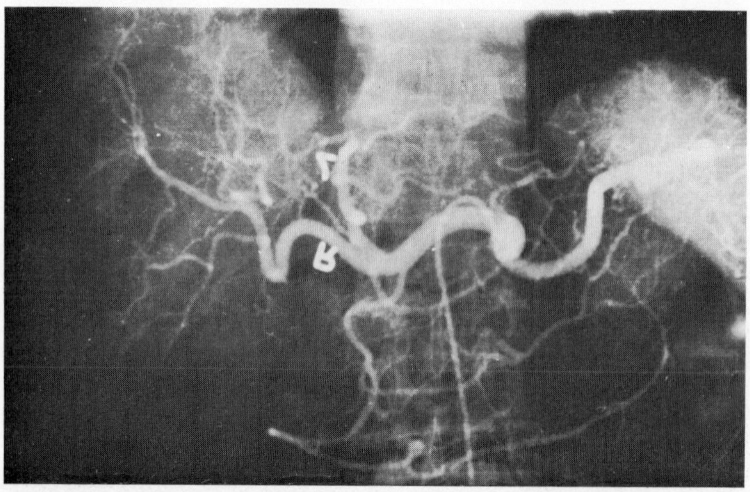

FIG. 9-5. Normal celiac arteriogram

with the multiple small venous tributaries entering it from the right caudate and quadrate lobes. With these veins on tension, fine silk ligatures can be passed around each of them individually and the veins cut between the ligatures. Whereas the number of these small venous branches is variable, anywhere from three to eight may be encountered before the major venous affluent from the liver is encountered close to the point where the vena cava passes through the diaphragm. Dissection in this area is probably the most critical part of the operation. One should be able to identify a large main right hepatic vein entering the vena cava at a slight angle and a second vein entering from the left lobe just medial to it. If only one large vein can be identified, the right and left hepatic veins have joined in a single trunk within the liver substance, and ultimate ligation of the right hepatic vein must be deferred until the liver has been partially transected and the point of junction identified. It is probably unnecessary to emphasize the catastrophe of damaging the hepatic vein, which will be the only source of outflow from the remaining liver tissue.

At this point attention is redirected towards the structures of the gastrohepatic ligament. The cystic duct and cystic artery are individually ligated and divided; the common duct is opened and probed to identify with certainty the major divisions of the biliary tract. The right hepatic duct, the right portal vein and the right hepatic artery are then securely ligated and divided. The operator can then return to the retroperitoneal area behind the liver and at this point ligate and divide the last and major right hepatic vein, presuming that the left hepatic vein has been satisfactorily identified and preserved. At this point, a line of demarcation will occur in the liver, identifying the devascularized portion that will include the right caudate and quadrate lobes. This line of vascular division between the lobes appears approximately 2 cm. to the right of the attachment of the round ligament. The liver capsule is then incised along the relatively avascular line of demarcation, and transection of the liver tissue itself can be carried out bluntly with the handle of a knife, permitting identification, clamping and division of the various biliary, portal and arterial structures that traverse the anatomic division. During the transection of the liver it is wise to have a metal probe through the opening in the common bile duct into the left bile duct since it may in its initial course pass very close to the planned line of transection. This easy method of identification will prevent inadvertent injury to this vital structure. As mentioned before, if it has not been possible to identify the right and left hepatic veins behind the liver, one must proceed cautiously through the liver tissue and identify their junction within the liver substance with certainty before dividing the right hepatic vein.

With the right lobe removed, there is relatively little bleeding from the cut surface once all the clamped structures have been ligated, and hemostasis can be secured easily by further identification of any residual bleeding points. At this point, a T-tube should be inserted in the common bile duct and the duct closed tightly around the tube. Colored

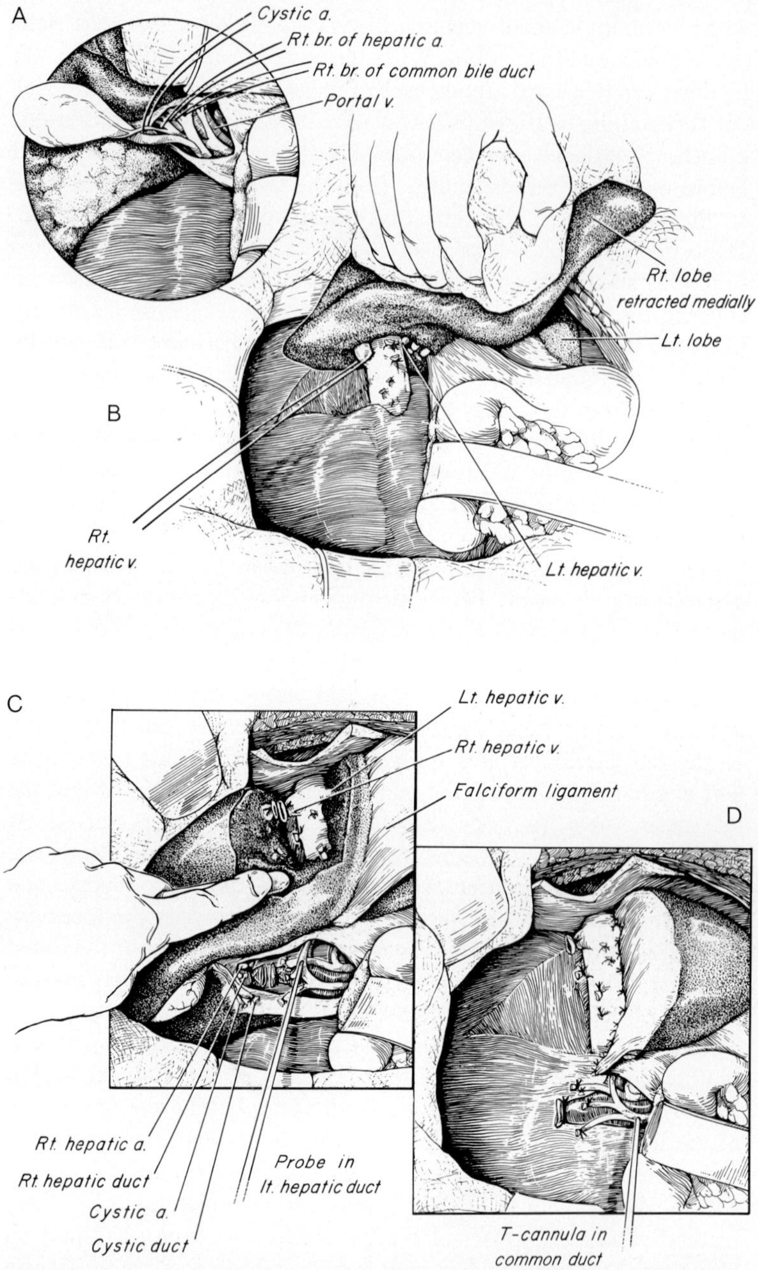

FIG. 9-6. Significant steps in right hepatic lobectomy: A, Identification and isolation of the appropriate structures in the gastrohepatic ligament. B, Retraction of the right lobe medially to expose the hepatic veins. C, Structures exposed after transection of liver and removal of right lobe. D, Completion of right hepatic lobectomy with falciform ligament used to reperitonealize the cut surface of the left lobe, with T-tube in common duct.

saline solution instilled into the T-tube will then identify any biliary radicles that had not been noted and ligated during the transection. This maneuver should secure against a postoperative bile leak that can be a very disturbing, prolonged and occasionally lethal complication. A satisfactory way to cover the raw surface of the liver is to detach the round ligament from the anterior abdominal wall with a section of the peritonealized attachment and suture it to the retroperitoneal tissue along the vena cava, thus providing a smooth and hemostatic covering.

A sump drain should be inserted in the right subphrenic area and the empty space left by removal of the large segment of liver, and an ordinary drain is inserted in the hepatorenal fossa. These drains and the T-tube are brought out through appropriate small stab wounds lateral to the incision. Closure of the thoracic wound, with a chest tube for drainage, and the abdominal component of the incision is accomplished according to standard techniques. Emphasis must be placed on the importance of using closely spaced retention sutures through all the layers of the abdominal incision, since the healing qualities of the patient following major hepatic resection are variable. The major points in the technique of right hepatic lobectomy are illustrated in Figure 9-6.

left hepatic lobectomy

A similar anatomic technique can be employed for removal of the left lobe of the liver. This is ordinarily not necessary because of the particular anatomic configuration of the left lobe, which tapers rapidly to a thinned-out segment of liver tissue. Under ordinary circumstances, after the coronary ligament has been divided and the left lobe mobilized, a satisfactory resection can be carried out by wedging the liver's tissue to permit very adequate closure with a series of interrupted mattress sutures. It is only when a tumor extends very close to the anatomic junction of the left lobe with the right caudate and quadrate lobes that the type of anatomic dissection described for right hepatic lobectomy may be required.

bibliography

hepatic tumors

Adam, Y. G., Huvos, A. G., and Hajdu, S. I.: Malignant vascular tumors of liver. Ann. Surg., *175:*375–383, 1972.

Alpert, M. E., and Davidson, C. S.: Mycotoxins. A possible cause of primary carcinoma of the liver. Amer. J. Med., *46:*325–329, 1969.

Alpert, M. E., Hutt, M. S. R., and Davidson, C. S.: Primary hepatoma in Uganda. A prospective clinical and epidemiologic study of forty-six patients. Amer. J. Med., *46:*794–802, 1969.

Altemeier, W. A., Schowengerdt, C. G., and Whiteley, D. H.: Abscesses of the liver: Surgical considerations. Arch. Surg., *101:*258–266, 1970.

Burdette, W. J. (Ed.): Primary Hepatoma. Salt Lake City, Utah, University of Utah Press, 1965, 150 pp.

Clifford, P., Linsell, C. A., and Timms, G. L. (Eds.): Cancer in Africa. Nairobi, Kenya, East African Publishing House, 1968, 458 pp.

Edmondson, H. A.: Tumors of the liver and intrahepatic bile ducts. *In* Atlas of Tumor Pathology. Section VII, fascicle 25. Washington, D.C., Armed Forces Institute of Pathology, 1958, 216 pp.

Henson, S. W., Jr., Gray, H. K., and Dockerty, M. B.: Benign tumors of the liver. I. Adenomas. Surg. Gynec. Obstet., *103:*23–30, 1956.

Kappel, D. A., and Miller, D. R.: Primary hepatic carcinoma. A review of thirty-seven patients. Amer. J. Surg., *124:*798–802, 1972.

Malt, R. A., Hershberg, R. A., and Miller, W. L.: Experience with benign tumors of the liver. Surg. Gynec. Obstet., *130:*285–291, 1970.

Suzuki, T., Sarumaru, S., Kawabe, K., and Honjo, I.: Study of vascularity of tumors of the liver. Surg. Gynec. Obstet., *134:*27–34, 1972.

Uganda Cancer Institute: Annual progress report 1971–1972. Contract No. PH 43-67-1343. Bethesda, Md., National Cancer Institute, 24 pp.

hepatic resection and other treatment

Almersjö, O., et al.: Evaluation of hepatic dearterialization in primary and secondary cancer of the liver. Amer. J. Surg., *124:*5–9, 1972.

Balasegaram, M.: Complete hepatic dearterialization for primary carcinoma of the liver. Report of twenty-four patients. Amer. J. Surg., *124:*340–345, 1972.

Brasfield, R. D., Bowden, L., and McPeak, C. J.: Major hepatic resection for malignant neoplasms of the liver. Ann. Surg., *176:*171–177, 1972.

Cady, B.: Hepatic arterial patency and complications after catheterization for infusion chemotherapy. Ann. Surg. (in press).

Cady, B., and Oberfield, R. A.: Regional infusion chemotherapy of hepatic metastases from colon carcinoma. Presented 5/23/73 at the Society of Surgery of Alimentary Tract Meeting, Americana Hotel, New York, N.Y. Amer. J. Surg., (to be published).

McDermott, W. V., Jr., and Ottinger, L. W.: Elective hepatic resection. Amer. J. Surg., *112:*376–381, 1966.

Mercadier, M. P., Clot, J.-P., and Cady, J.-P.: Right hepatectomy in the treatment of liver trauma. Amer. J. Surg., *124:*353–358, 1972.

Watkins, E., Jr., Khazei, A. M., and Nahra, K. S.: Surgical basis for arterial infusion chemotherapy of disseminated carcinoma of the liver. Surg. Gynec. Obstet., *130:*581–605, 1970.

Metabolic Changes and Regeneration following Hepatic Resection

CHAPTER 10

Surgery involving the removal of only small segments of the liver does not entail any particular problems relating to hepatic function. The changes to be described in the subsequent paragraphs relate primarily to the procedure of right hepatic lobectomy, which entails removal of approximately 85 per cent of functioning liver tissue. In one of our patients it was necessary, in order to encompass the tumor, to remove the medial segment of the left lobe as well, by identifying the further subdivisions of the vascular and biliary arborizations. This case was of particular interest because certainly no more than 10 per cent of functioning liver tissue remained, indicating the enormous reserve in hepatic function that exists, the rapid restoration of adequate function and the subsequent regeneration within six months to a liver mass approximating the normal size (Fig. 10-1).

carbohydrate metabolism

Adequate studies of glucose metabolism following major hepatic lobectomy have not been carried out because of the risk of sudden and possibly fatal hypoglycemia that may occur if continuous, slow infusion of 10 per cent glucose is not administered throughout the first 48 hours. It is clear from our own observations, however, that hypoglycemia is an unpredictable but definite threat during the immediate postoperative phase but can be easily controlled by glucose infusions.

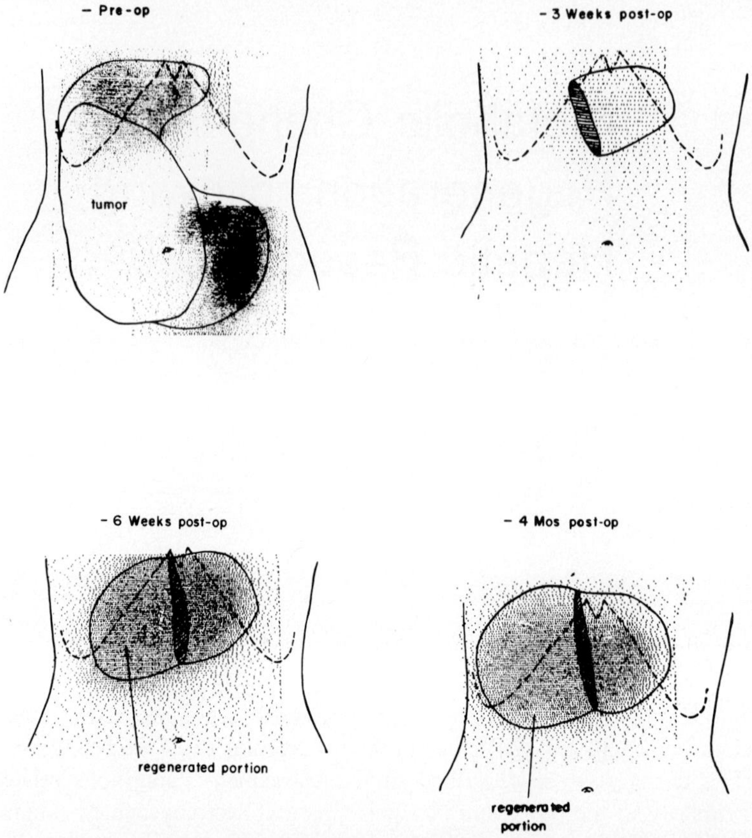

FIG. 10-1. Sequential scintiscans indicating the rate of hepatic regeneration after 90 per cent resection. (Reproduced from McDermott, W. V., Jr., et al.: Major Hepatic Resection: Diagnostic Techniques and Metabolic Problems. Surgery *54:* 56–66, 1963, with permission of the Publishers)

protein metabolism

From the information available at the present time, it would appear that the liver is the source of all the plasma albumin, fibrinogen and most of the globulin, and, therefore, one might expect considerable derangement in protein metabolism following major hepatic resection. Without reviewing all the available information on changes after total or partial hepatectomy in various types of laboratory animals, a consistent pattern emerges in man following right hepatic lobectomy, as noted from our own studies and those reported by Pack and Molander. The most consistent and certainly the most significant change is the progressive drop in the serum albumin levels during the first seven to ten days after resection. Whether this is caused by the initial inability of the small amount of residual liver to cope with the ordinary catabolic demands of the body after a major operative procedure, or whether it is caused more specifically by a tremendously increased demand for protein related to the process of regeneration within the residual liver, is not entirely clear at the present time. In addition, there are considerable individual variations in the degree of decrease in serum albumin levels that are, of course, related to the amount of residual liver and apparently also to the age of the patient. Regardless, there is a demonstrable need for the administration of varying amounts of human serum albumin, particularly during the first postoperative week. On the average, our patients have required between 100 and 200 gm. of parenterally administered albumin to maintain a reasonable level of serum albumin and to prevent the tremendous shifts in fluid and electrolyte balance that occur if a significant fall in the intravascular osmotic pressure is permitted to develop. From the point of view of the clinical management of the postresection patient, the importance of careful monitoring of protein levels cannot be overemphasized. At 10 to 12 days after operation, stabilization seems to occur, although in individual cases a continued drift downward has been noted and continued supplementation required.

There has been no consistent fall in globulin levels, and electrophoretic patterns have not varied consistently except for minor changes that have been observed in the alpha-2 globulin.

Fibrinogen, which has a biologic half-life of about 12 hours, will decrease to varying degrees during the first postoperative week. Unless this period is accompanied by some additional postoperative problem such as massive hemorrhage or a consumptive coagulopathy, the changes are not clinically significant and have no serious effect on the coagulation mechanism.

bilirubin metabolism

Bilirubinemia of a varying degree has been a consistent finding after major hepatic resection. In those patients in whom a T-tube permits measurement of the bile output, the total volume during the first 24 hour period is less than 100 cc. This gradually increases towards normal levels over the subsequent seven to ten days. This decrease in bile outflow is accompanied by bilirubinemia; bilirubin may on occasion reach levels over 30 mg. per 100 ml., and, of course, obvious clinical jaundice is a frequent accompaniment. The pattern in terms of fractionation of bilirubin level is that of obstructive type of jaundice, and the alkaline phosphatase levels are concomitantly elevated. Scintiscans with technetium are consistent with intrahepatic cholestatic jaundice, and the normal pattern on cholangiography would also indicate that this is not an obstructive mechanism involving the extrahepatic biliary tree. One could postulate that the sudden diversion of the total portal inflow to a small residual segment of liver could cause initial hepatic congestion and compression of the bile canaliculi; this supposition is supported by the transient portal hypertension that consistently occurs in the immediate postresection period. Regardless of the pathogenesis of this jaundice and bilirubinemia, the surgeon can be reassured that normal levels will be re-established gradually during the postoperative period, and we have never seen permanent elevations remain beyond several weeks. *Prothrombin time* is another evidence of the abnormalities in synthetic function after major hepatic resection. The prothrombin levels are depressed during the postoperative phase despite parenteral administration of vitamin K. This depression consistently falls to the range of 30 per cent of normal and remains there for several weeks but is not accompanied by any clinical disorder in the clotting mechanism.

lipid metabolism

Following major hepatic resection in man, there is a fall in the level of cholesterol, with almost complete absence of esterification, and in the phospholipids, triglycerides and nonesterified fatty acids. Although there is usually a restoration to normal blood levels within three weeks, the kinetics are interesting in that the nonesterified fatty acids, after an initial fall in the first few days, show a rapid rise to as high as 2,500 mEq. per L. preceding the subsequent and more gradual rise in the triglycerides, phospholipids and cholesterol (Fig. 10-2C). Since these other dramatic changes are not apparently accompanied by any clinical abnormality, the observations are primarily of academic interest.

serum enzymes

Although varying elevations in glutamic oxaloacetic transaminase, glutamic pyruvic transaminase and lactic dehydrogenase are seen after partial hepatectomy in man and in laboratory animals, the degree of change does not coincide with the extent of the hepatic resection and may well reflect individual variations in the amount of devitalized liver tissue left *in situ* after resection.

blood coagulation

Reference has already been made to the increased prothrombin time and the decreased fibrinogen level. Reports from Bengmark and his associates have referred to depressions in factors II, V, VII and X. *Decrease in platelets* and an occasional increase in *fibrinolysis* do not seem consistently related to hepatic resection, and the changes are no more pronounced than may be seen after any major surgical procedure. From the clinical point of view, one might say that there are no clinically significant or dangerous changes in the coagulating mechanism of the blood relative to the loss of 80 per cent or more of functioning hepatic tissue unless serious complications such as gram-negative septicemia, gastrointestinal hemorrhage or other postoperative complications develop. Because of the ordinary requirement of 4 to 10 units of blood during the operative procedure, it has been our custom to replace at least one half of the demonstrable blood loss with units that have been drawn less than 48 hours prior to surgery. With these simple precautions, no major problems related to the blood clotting mechanism have been encountered.

summary

The clinically significant metabolic changes that occur after major hepatic resection are: (1) a decrease in bile flow and bilirubinemia during the two to three weeks following operation; (2) variable hypoglycemia during the first 48 hours; (3) a decrease in prothrombin time to about 30 per cent of normal; (4) a decrease in serum albumin levels to the degree that parenteral support with human serum albumin is usually required to support the intravascular osmotic pressure.

These changes are illustrated in the metabolic charts reproduced in Figure 10-2 (A to C).

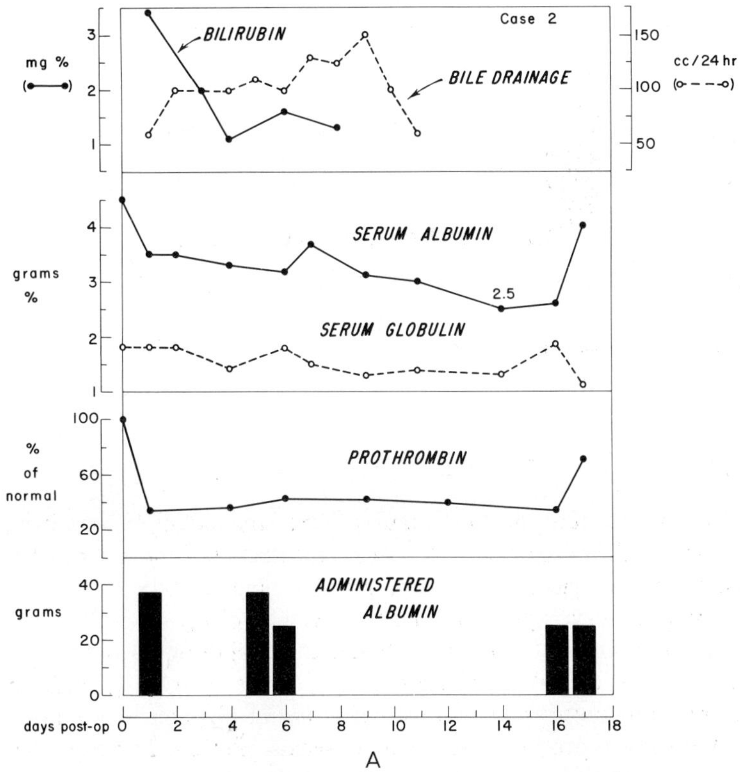

FIG. 10-2. A, B, and C. Metabolic changes following major hepatic resection. (Reproduced from McDermott, W. V., Jr., et al.: Major Hepatic Resection: Diagnostic Techniques and Metabolic Problems. Surgery, 54:56–66, 1963, with permission of the Publishers)

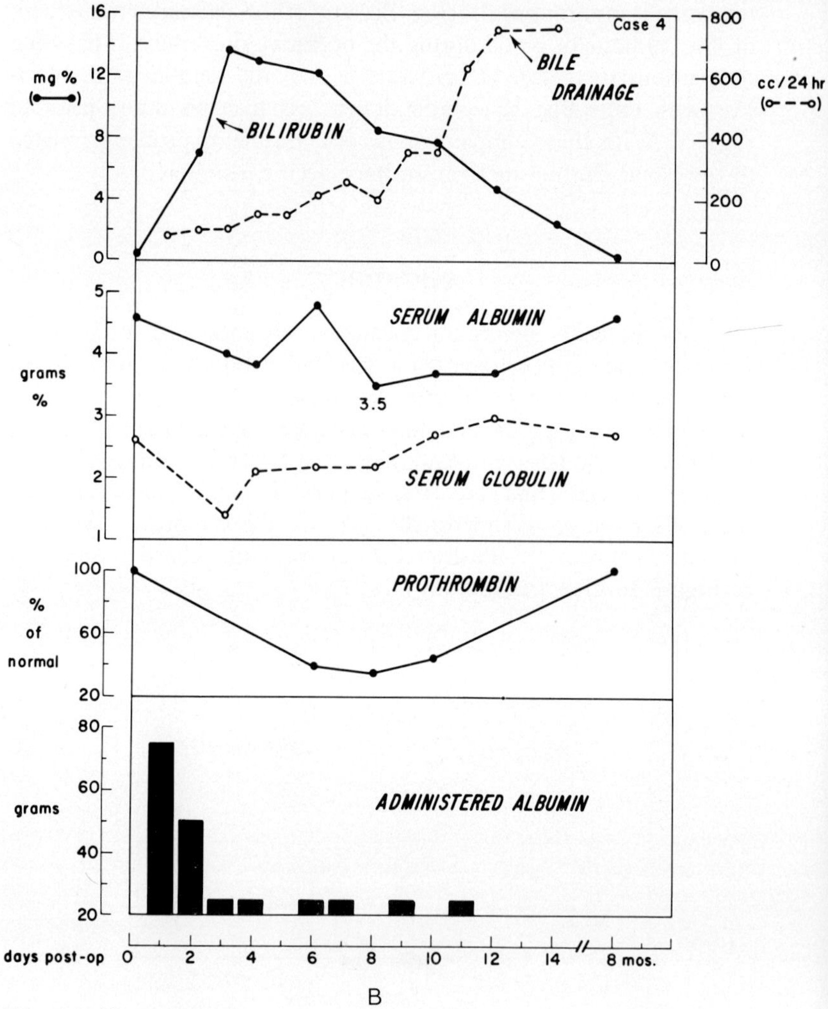

FIG. 10-2. (Continued)

hepatic regeneration

Since the turn of the century, increasing attention has been focused on the phenomenon of hepatic regeneration, although the term itself may be inaccurate, and the process might best be referred to as compensatory hyperplasia and hypertrophy of the liver.

Almost invariably an introduction to this subject refers to the myth in which the Titans' punishment of Prometheus for stealing fire from Olympus involved the repetitive devouring of his liver by a vulture and equally repetitive restoration. It seems unlikely, however, that the original construction of the myth was based on a recognition of the remarkable regenerative capacity of the liver but rather to familiarity, even at that time, with the intermittent agony of the symptoms of biliary colic.

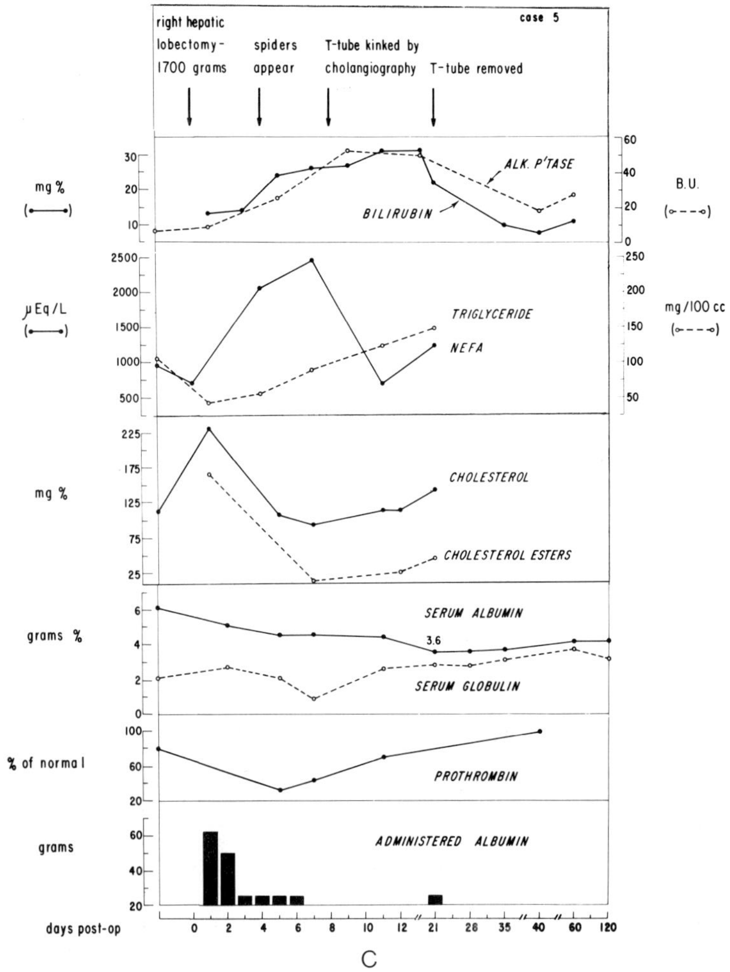

FIG. 10-2. (Continued)

Regardless of the validity of the reference point to Prometheus, the investigation of this phenomenon, which is common to most mammalian species, has developed its own mythology as well as a hard core of incontrovertible and soundly based scientific observation.

In two superb review articles, Bucher has summarized the morphologic, physiologic and biochemical studies that have been done over the past half century in this fascinating area, and for anything more extensive than the superficial view given here, the reader is referred to these articles, both for their intrinsic analytic and synthetic value and for the extensive bibliography that has been compiled.

Although our primary interest may be concerned with the phenomenon of hepatic regeneration in man as it occurs after major hepatic resection, much of our information must be extrapolated from the extensive studies done on other mammalian organisms. The rapidity of the process varies with the species; in the rat, regeneration is probably complete within three weeks, in the dog within ten weeks and in man within about four months. Although the pace may vary, the sequence of events, as compiled so well from studies in the rat, is probably similar in all species. Normally, the hepatocyte is a long lived cell, and proliferative activity in the normal adult liver, as indicated by mitotic activity, is low. Following resection of more than two thirds of the liver (the common experimental preparation in the rat), a tremendous burst of proliferative activity, as indicated by the incorporation of radioactive precursors into DNA, occurs within 24 hours. Initially, the labeled nuclei are concentrated in the peripheral areas of the hepatic lobule but rapidly extend centrally, eventually

TABLE 10-1. Sequence of Morphologic Changes Following Hepatic Resection in the Rat

Time after hepatectomy	
30 minutes	Dispersion of basophilic bodies of the cytoplasm observed in cells at the periphery of the lobule and gradually spreading to the center during the ensuing 8 hours. Disaggregation of the endoplasmic reticulum, loss of membranes and dispersion of ribonucleoprotein particles (ribosomes)
2–3 hours	Cytoplasmic inclusions appear, and slightly later, accumulations of lipid
6–10 hours	Loss of glycogen, falling to very low levels by 10 hours and remaining low for several days
12 hours	Perceptible increase in the size of cells, nuclei and nucleoli, which becomes maximal in 24 hours when mitosis begins
16–18 hours	Endoplasmic reticulum begins to re-form, characteristically in close contact with groups of mitochondria
18–24 hours	Rapid increase in proliferative activity as indicated by the incorporation of radioactive precursors into DNA. Initially, labeled nuclei are concentrated in periportal areas, later extending towards the central vein and then becoming randomly distributed
24–30 hours	Mitotic activity follows DNA labeling by 6 to 8 hours and exhibits a similar pattern of distribution within the lobule
30–72 hours	This period includes a sharp peak in both DNA and mitotic activity, both of which then fall off rapidly
3–18 days	The rapid growth phase falls off after the third day, and regeneration slowly proceeds to completion within 3 weeks

becoming distributed throughout the entire lobule. A more exact description of the sequence of events after resection is given in Table 10-1. The extraordinary burst of activity that follows within the first 48 hours after hepatic resection subsides after the third day, and the total regenerative process gradually evolves, reaching completion within about three weeks. The degree of this proliferative activity is influenced directly by the amount of liver removed, and if less than a third of the liver is resected, no demonstrable evidence of growth stimulus appears.

Information available on the regenerative response in man must of necessity be incomplete and fortuitous. From the metabolic patterns, "second look" operations, scintiscans, selective arteriography and postmortem material, a certain reasonable pattern of the events as they occur in man can be deduced. In terms of *metabolic changes,* as already described, restoration of adequate function occurs within three weeks, but some biochemical abnormalities persist for as long as four months. Pack and his associates, in second look laparotomies in four patients, have described the rounded, spherical form that the regenerated human liver takes and have pointed out that it can usually be palpated as a smooth mass in the epigastrium, sometimes confused with recurrent cancer. From these data and from a typical series of sequential scintiscans (Fig. 10-1), it would certainly appear that the regenerative process, taking approximately four months in man, is similar to that which has been so well defined in the rat. The gross appearance of a human liver after full regeneration is shown in Figure 10-3. This postmortem specimen came from a patient who recovered

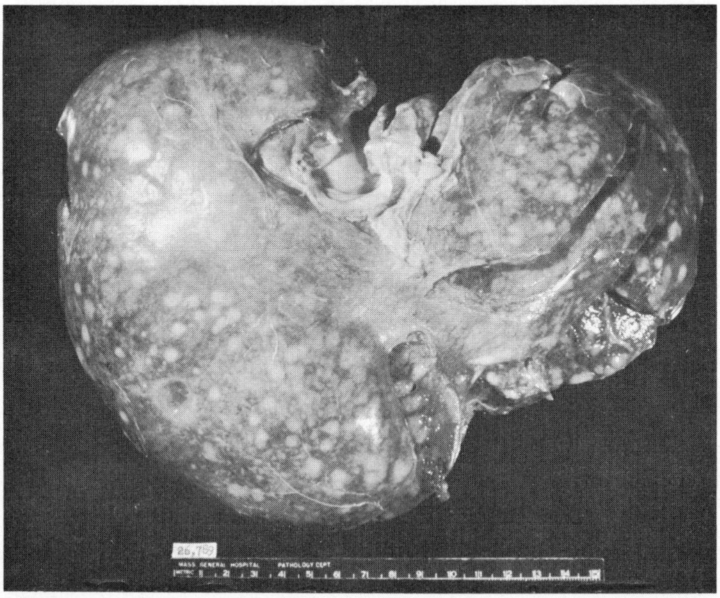

FIG. 10-3. The gross appearance of a human liver three years after right hepatic lobectomy for a benign tumor. Cause of death was carcinoma of the pancreas with liver metastases.

uneventfully from a right hepatic lobectomy for a benign tumor only to die three years later of carcinoma of the pancreas with liver metastases.

Regulatory mechanisms concerned with hepatic regeneration have been the subject of intensive study. Obviously one of the key questions relating to this remarkable phenomenon of rapid hepatic regeneration after resection has been the nature of the forces involved in the initiation and cessation of the process. As referred to previously, the regenerative process is directly related to the amount of liver removed, and there is a certain amount of organ specificity inasmuch as the main impact is on the liver cells, although there has been evidence presented that indicates some increased mitotic activity in several extrahepatic tissues and some increased growth of implanted tumors. In the early studies, a great deal of stress was laid on the increase in portal pressure and relative blood flow to the residual segment of liver, and it was demonstrated by Bollman and by Child that diversion of the portal blood through an Eck fistula was attended by a very significant loss in the ability of the liver to regenerate after resection. Subsequent studies concerned with the regulatory mechanisms have tended to downgrade the importance of blood flow and assign a permissive rather than a direct effect of flow on hepatic regeneration.

The search for humoral factors has been the subject of innumerable, ingenious experimental designs, but legitimate controversy still exists in this area. To quote Bucher, "It remains unsettled whether growth is normally held in check by inhibitors that disappear during regeneration or whether an active stimulus develops. Although growth inhibitors which have blocked mitosis of the cells in tissue culture are extractable from normal liver, their relation to regeneration is unknown." Although the evidence is conflicting, there certainly is important evidence from studies on subcutaneous autoimplants of liver, parabiotic rats and tissue cultures that some type of humoral control over the regenerative process does exist. In fact, this whole area still presents a tremendous challenge to the ingenious and imaginative investigator, and the immense importance of the information to be gathered extends far beyond the scope of the phenomenon of hepatic regeneration itself.

bibliography

regeneration of liver

Bucher, N. L. R.: Regeneration of mammalian liver. Int. Rev. Cytol., *15:* 245-300, 1963.

Bucher, N. L. R.: Experimental aspects of hepatic regeneration. New Eng. J. Med., *277:*686-696; 738-746, 1967.

Child, C. G., III, Barr, D., Holswade, G. R., and Harrison, C. S.: Liver regeneration following portacaval transposition in dogs. Ann. Surg., *138:*600-608, 1953.

Goldsmith, H. S., and Castillo, J.: Direct vascular implantation of liver for hepatic regeneration after interruption of the portal vein and hepatic artery. Amer. J. Surg., *121:*100–104, 1971.

Grindlay, J. H., and Bollman, J. L.: Regeneration of the liver in the dog after partial hepatectomy. Surg. Gynec. Obstet., *94:*491–496, 1952.

Islami, A. H., Pack, G. T., and Hubbard, J. C.: The humoral factor in regeneration of the liver in parabiotic rats. Surg. Gynec. Obstet., *108:* 549–554, 1959.

Max, M. H., Price, J. B., Jr., Takeshige, K., and Voorhees, A. B., Jr.: The role of factors of portal origin in modifying hepatic regeneration. J. Surg. Res., *12:*120–123, 1972.

Monaco, A. P., Hallgrimsson, J., and McDermott, W. V., Jr.: Multiple adenoma (hamartoma) of the liver treated by subtotal (90%) resection: Morphological and functional studies of regeneration. Ann. Surg., *159:* 513–519, 1964.

Pack, G. T., Islami, A. H., Hubbard, J. C., and Brasfield, R. D.: Regeneration of human liver after major hepatectomy. Surgery, *52:*617–623, 1962.

Rabinovici, N., and Vardi, J.: The effect of regeneration on the hemodynamics of the cirrhotic liver after hepatectomy. Surg. Gynec. Obstet., *116:*533–538, 1963.

Wexler, M., et al.: Regeneration and maintenance of integrity of canine liver. The role of arterial, portal, and systemic venous blood. Arch. Surg., *101:*267–276, 1970.

postresection metabolism

Conn, R.: Right hepatic lobectomy in children. Amer. J. Surg., *118:*512–516, 1969.

McDermott, W. V., Jr., Greenberger, N. J., Isselbacher, K. J., and Weber, A. L.: Major hepatic resection: Diagnostic techniques and metabolic problems. Surgery, *54:*56–66, 1963.

Nikaidoh, H., Boggs, J., and Swenson, O.: Liver tumors in infants and children. Clinical and pathological analysis of 22 cases. Arch. Surg., *101:*245–257, 1970.

Pack, G. T., and Molander, D. W.: Metabolism before and after hepatic lobectomy for cancer. Studies in twenty-three patients. Arch. Surg., *80:*685–692, 1960.

Transplantation of the Liver and Auxiliary Support

CHAPTER 11

Of all the organs in which experimental and clinical efforts at transplantation have been directed, the liver is certainly the most complicated from the metabolic point of view and the most difficult from the technical aspects of the surgery. There are three major directions in which remarkable progress has been made during the past decade. Through the pioneering work of Starzl and others, orthotopic transplantation has become a clinical reality. In patients whose disease process does not require removal of the liver, heterotopic transplantation has been attempted, and a number of other forms of auxiliary liver support have been tested (Table 11-1). Since the problems in these three areas are so different, they will be considered under separate headings.

orthotopic liver transplantation

The technical, metabolic and immunologic problems concerned with orthotopic transplantation of the liver have recently been reviewed extensively by Starzl, and it seems redundant to comment upon the experimental and clinical material that he has so well presented. Certainly orthotopic transplantation in man has become a feasible procedure, and immediate success in this area has been achieved by a number of surgeons. In terms of patient salvage and long term survival, however, the outlook at the moment is far from encouraging. The 1971 report from the ACS/NIH Organ Transplant Registry shows that of 102 orthotopic liver transplants attempted over the past eight years, there were at that time (January 1971) only 12

TABLE 11-1. Liver Transplantation and Auxiliary Liver Support

- I. Liver transplantation
  - A. Orthotopic allograft
  - B. Auxiliary heterotopic liver transplant
    - 1. Human (whole or partial)
    - 2. Primate
- II. Exchange (fresh whole blood or plasma)
- III. Dialysis (hemodialysis or peritoneal dialysis)
- IV. Cross circulation (human or primate)
- V. *Ex vivo* auxiliary liver (pig, calf etc.)

survivors; the longest survivor was living and well at 29 months after his transplant. Causes of immediate failure have included peritonitis, vascular thrombosis, pneumonia, hemorrhage and a number of other immediate postoperative problems. The long term failures are related to rejection of the graft, infection during an immunosuppressive program and recurrence of malignant disease. In fact, the high incidence of recurrence after removal of the liver for malignant disease has raised the serious question whether the required immunosuppression interferes so much with the surveillance mechanism that hepatectomy and transplantation for cancer are contraindicated. Of the 46 total hepatectomies with orthotopic transplantation carried out for cancer, 14 patients survived more than 90 days, and of these 14, six died of metastatic disease; seven patients died of other causes, and one was still alive at 358 days without evidence of recurrent disease. Certainly these limited data are not sufficient to answer the question definitively. The high percentage of patients who did develop early metastatic disease would suggest that immunosuppression may contribute to early seeding and recurrence. On the other hand, the fact that one patient has survived nearly a year on a continuous immunosuppressive regimen might lend some encouragement to continuing this approach to otherwise inoperable and incurable cancer. Obviously, however, optimism in this area must be guarded, and the limited number of satisfactory results have occurred in nonmalignant disease of the liver, particularly in cases of biliary atresia. These observations lead to a consideration of other approaches to nonmalignant disease of the liver.

heterotopic liver transplantation

There is obvious appeal in the concept of a heterotopically implanted liver in the treatment of conditions that would not, of necessity, require removal of the donor liver to effect cure or amelioration. Biliary atresia might be one of these conditions, although even if problems in bilirubin metabolism could be controlled by permanent heterotopically implanted liver, one might still face the long term problems of biliary cirrhosis and the attendant portal hypertension. Even more appealing is the concept of the use of an auxiliary liver in the treatment of fulminant hepatic failure in which one might reasonably anticipate the possibility of ultimate recovery of the host liver and removal of the transplanted donor liver. The use of the auxiliary *ex vivo* perfused pig liver and other measures of temporary support lend some credence to this hypothesis. The various methods that have been employed to provide temporary support for the organism with fulminant hepatic failure will be described later. Relative to the problem of auxiliary liver transplantation, one might say that other *ex vivo* forms of support have been temporary or intermittent in nature and in general have not carried the functionally anhepatic host for a sufficiently long period to observe any significant degree of hepatic regeneration. One might reasonably ask if any regeneration at all could be expected in the type of lethal, fulminant hepatic failure one sees occasionally with viral hepatitis, alcoholic hepatitis or halothane-induced hepatic necrosis, the three major causes of the type of hepatic failure that we are considering. Because of the known capacity of the liver for regeneration after extensive resection or diffuse metabolic injury, it is not unreasonable to explore this avenue of treatment since the syndrome itself with present methods of treatment carries a mortality of close to 90 per cent if one uses strict criteria employed by Trey. The technical and metabolic problems concerned with heterotopic transplantation of the liver can be summarized as follows, and each problem will be considered separately.

hepatotrophic factors in portal blood

There is a considerable body of experimental evidence that would suggest that portal blood carries factors essential for maximal liver function and for regeneration. Innumerable experimental studies have been done in an attempt to clarify this still controversial problem, but as yet it remains an unsettled question. Certainly with diversion of portal blood from the normal liver there is subsequent atrophy and failure of the normal regenerative process that occurs after partial hepatic resection. On the other hand, if systemic venous blood is diverted to the liver by portacaval transposition, significant atrophy does not occur, and regeneration takes place at a near normal rate and degree. With this preparation, however, portal blood still reaches the liver since it is diverted into the systemic circulation via the portacaval shunt. Almost every experimental study comes down finally to the fact that, regardless of the preparation, there still exists the possibility of portal blood reaching the liver through other than normal channels.

The ultimate and possibly conclusive experiment has not yet been done; this would entail a totally eviscerated animal devoid of splanchnic blood and maintained nutritionally and metabolically in a near normal state. Only with this total absence of a splanchnic circulation and any source of portal blood could the appropriate studies be done to determine whether maintenance and regeneration of the normal liver can occur in the total absence of the suggested hepatotrophic factors. Regardless of the academic outcome of this controversial point, there is sufficient evidence extant to indicate that portal blood directly perfusing a heterotopically transplanted liver is not absolutely essential for its maintenance and growth.

competitive inhibition of the graft with the host and subsequent graft atrophy

In the presence of a normally functioning liver a transplanted homograft will undergo progressive atrophy and loss of function. Varying experimental preparations have been designed to demonstrate quite conclusively that when sufficient damage has been done to the host liver—through bile duct ligation, partial devascularization or extensive resection—a liver homograft will function and show regeneration and growth. Under clinical conditions of severe liver damage, therefore, one might expect that a satisfactorily transplanted liver homograft could function, grow and temporarily support the functionally anhepatic host.

assessment of donor liver function

If one is projecting a temporary transplanted auxiliary liver, the problem arises as the host recovers whether it is the regenerated host liver or the functioning auxiliary liver that is supporting the organism. By monitoring haptoglobins which are different for the two livers, it should be possible to determine the degree of regeneration of the host liver and to estimate the optimal point at which the temporarily transplanted liver could be removed safely. One, of course, faces then the theoretic problem whether or not the presence of a heterotopically implanted homograft would suppress by reverse inhibition the expected regeneration of the damaged host liver. Certainly this particular question has not been defined satisfactorily and probably will not be until sufficient satisfactory clinical experience has been gained.

technical problems

Despite a moderate amount of both experimental and clinical experience, the ideal technical procedure for the auxiliary transplant has not been defined. The general categories of auxiliary transplants have been defined by Slapak and colleagues as shown in Figure 11-1. Various modifications in each of these four categories have been attempted, but these generally portray the major technical differences in the various preparations.

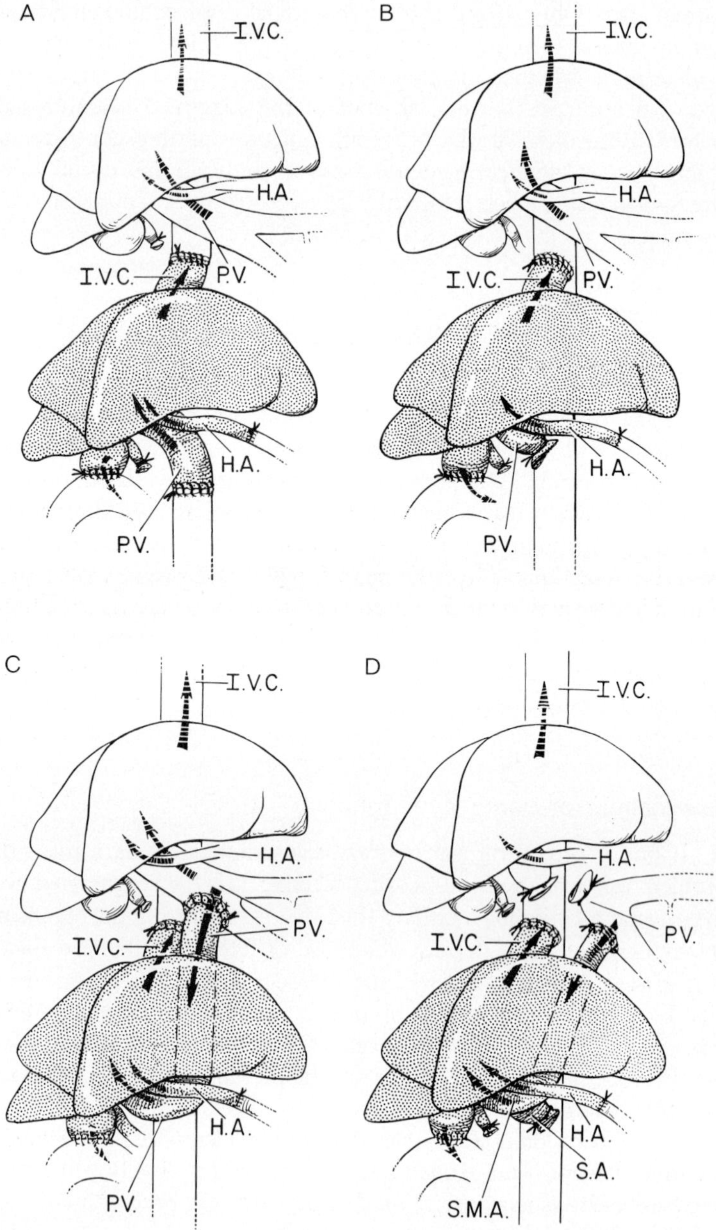

FIG. 11-1. A–D, Various types of vascular and biliary reconstructions used in auxiliary liver transplant

With either small vessel anastomoses or low flow venous connections, there is the considerable risk of thrombosis, and this has occurred in most of the procedures employed to date in a relatively high percentage of the cases. Normally the flow through the venous outflow is maintained by the high inflow pressures from the combined arterial and portal circulation, by the sucking effect of respiration and diaphragmatic motion and by the hemodynamic effects of the streaming of caval blood by the orifices of the hepatic veins; all of these factors are not operable in most of the techniques of heterotopic transplant. Arterialization of the portal vein to provide inflow may provide a solution to thrombosis of the channels supplying the auxiliary liver, but experience has demonstrated that long term success with this particular approach is dependent on control of pressure with a Teflon cuff to prevent the adverse effects of high pressure blood entering the portal bed in the liver.

In summary, the ideal technical procedure for auxiliary liver transplant is not immediately discernible, but there is little doubt that these problems can be worked out if the other aspects of the problem are satisfactorily defined.

space

Transplantation of an additional large organ such as the liver into the abdominal cavity creates a space problem. Ideally, a liver from a child cadaver donor should be used, but these are obviously not readily available. Hemihepatectomy from a living donor has been suggested but not attempted, and the risk of such a procedure raises moral and ethical questions. Partial resection of a donor liver during perfusion and cooling has been used experimentally by us and by others and may have ultimate clinical application. The ideal location for an auxiliary transplant would probably be the iliac fossa and pelvis, but other intra-abdominal sites have been tried in experimental models.

procurement

The problem of procuring a satisfactory liver for a patient in fulminant hepatic failure involves the obvious fact that it is very unlikely that a satisfactory cadaver donor will be immediately available at the time of the acute liver crisis. One faces, therefore, the choice of achieving a goal of long term preservation of a donor liver, of using partial hepatic resection in a volunteer donor or of employing a xenograft, preferably from one of the primate species. Efforts at long term preservation of the liver have not to date been crowned with any high degree of success, and until this proves feasible, one must look to one of the other possibilities. The question of partial hepatic resection from a volunteer donor for transplantation to a temporarily anhepatic host involves a number of moral and ethical questions. Certainly this procedure is considerably more dangerous for the donor than the nephrectomy employed on the volunteer donor for a kidney transplant. In addition, technical problems of hemostasis and prevention of biliary leaks in the partial transplant are formidable although probably not insurmountable. Clearly, attention at this particular point should be and has been directed to the use of a xenograft whereby a small, adequately perfused and normal primate liver could be removed electively and transplanted intact into the anhepatic recipient. Were it not for the very serious immunologic problems and the intense rejection that so commonly occur when one crosses species in the use of xenografts, this particular approach would seem ideal. With increased knowledge of immunosuppression, however, the use of a xenograft for an auxiliary heterotopic liver transplant may well be feasible, particularly from certain types of primates that do not cross react with man as vigorously as other species.

clinical results

The record of auxiliary liver grafts in man to date has not been encouraging. As of the spring of 1971, 34 heterografts had been utilized, but only one functioned for more than a few weeks, and the patient in this one temporary success died from sepsis after 240 days. Even this period is encouraging, however, and might indicate that, if the problems as outlined above could be solved progressively, a temporarily implanted xenograft as an auxiliary liver might prove the solution to the otherwise fatal cases of fulminant hepatic failure.

ex vivo liver support

Efforts to sustain the liver in an *ex vivo* state by a perfusion system date back more than 100 years and are summarized in Table 11-2. Based on decades of experimental work, a number of ingenious and sometimes effective methods have been employed to support patients through a period of hepatic failure. These will be discussed under general headings below. For the most part, they have not been successful because the effect, if any, is usually temporary and intermittent, and none of the methods employed has been able to carry a patient through a prolonged anhepatic phase. Of all those utilized, exchange transfusion has probably been the most effective because of its sim-

TABLE 11-2. Evolution of Methods of Sustaining an *Ex Vivo* Liver by Organ Perfusion

1855 Claude Bernard—canine	1955 Young and Prudden—rodent
1926 Lamp and Mehes—feline	1960 Shoemaker—canine
1926 Rössler—canine	1960 Ostasherer—rodent
1932 Baur—canine	1961 Chapman—bovine
1934 Fiessinger—canine	1961 Eiseman—porcine
1936 Lundsgaard—feline—canine	1961 Kestens and McDermott—canine
1951 Brauer—rodent	1961 Healey—canine
1951 Miller—rodent	1962 Condon—bovine
1952 Werthessen and Schwenk—por.	1962 Huston—canine
1953 Andrews	1963 Mortimore—rodent
1954 Kruhófer and Muntz—feline	1963 Evans—rodent
1963 Munsch and Eiseman—canine	

plicity, its ease of repetition and its immediate although not very prolonged effect in altering the metabolic state of the patient in fulminant hepatic failure.

hemodialysis

This particular technique has not proved to be as effective in liver failure as it has demonstrably been in acute and chronic renal failure. While toxic metabolites may be removed by this technique, the liver is so much more complicated a biochemical factory than the kidney that it is not surprising that the disparity in results in these different examples of organ failure is so striking. In severe hepatic failure, one must not only remove abnormal and toxic metabolic products but must also substitute a number of factors ordinarily synthesized by the liver that are essential to the organism. Techniques of hemodialysis that have been employed are varied and include one identical to that used in renal dialysis, various methods of exchange through anion exchange column and peritoneal dialysis. All these variations are quite effective in removing ammonia from the blood, but it is quite clear that ammonia toxicity is only one of the many severe metabolic disorders that occur in fulminant hepatic failure. In exogenous encephalopathy in which hyperammoniemia is a major factor accounting for the central nervous system disorder, techniques of dialysis can be quite effective but are usually not necessary since other methods of management, which are described elsewhere, have been very satisfactorily utilized.

ex vivo liver perfusion

During the past few years, a number of groups have explored the possibility of perfusing the blood of a patient dying from fulminant hepatic failure through the liver of another mammalian organism. The pig and the calf have been the most commonly used species in procuring the liver for *ex vivo* perfusion, and the results in both, although temporarily gratifying on occasions, have not led to any significant numbers of permanent cures. In Figures 11-2 and 11-3 are shown the stages in preparation of the porcine liver and the system employed by our own group in exploring this method of treatment. Like others, we have seen many examples of dramatic improvement after a prolonged period of *ex vivo* liver perfusion, but invariably relapse has occurred, and three weeks is the longest we have been able to maintain a patient with widespread hepatic necrosis. In our own series death has ultimately occurred primarily because of invasive sepsis or, more commonly, from a terminal episode of gastrointestinal hemorrhage from multiple gastric erosions. Even after multiple, intermittent *ex vivo* perfusions we have been unable to detect any antibodies even though increasing levels of pig albumin and alpha-1 and -2 globulins have been demonstrated in the blood of the patients treated by this

STAGES OF CLINICAL PORCINE LIVER PERFUSION

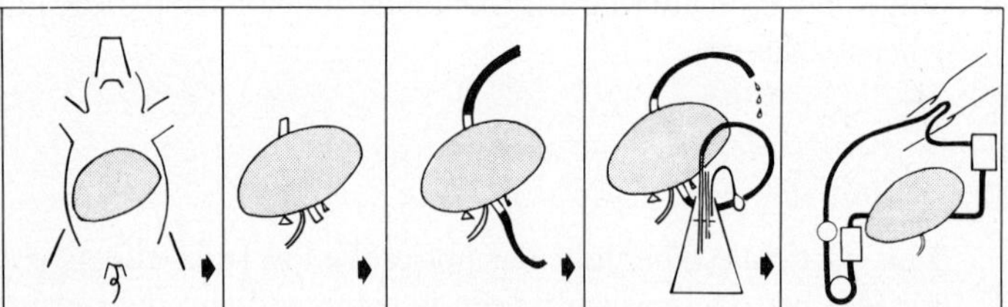

	PREPARATION	IN VIVO DISSECTION	EXCISION	CANNULATION	FLUSHING	EX VIVO PERFUSION
CURRENT ADJUNCTS	Antibiotics Purina Pig Chow	Monitoring Heparinization Hemodilution Buffering	Dispatch Atraumatic Manipulation	Air Embolus Mechanical Obstruction	Oxygen Heparinization Buffering Hypothermia → Normothermia	Portal Vein, alone
CONCEIVABLE ADJUNCTS	Glycogen Loading	Hypothermia Adrenergic and Metabolic Block Hyperbaria		Sealing of Capsule		Portal V. and Hepatic Art. Inflow Oxygenation Heat Exchanger Outflow Oxygenation

← - - - - - - - ←—— *ISCHEMIA* ——→

←—— *STORAGE* ——→

FIG. 11-2. Preparation of porcine liver for *ex vivo* auxiliary perfusion

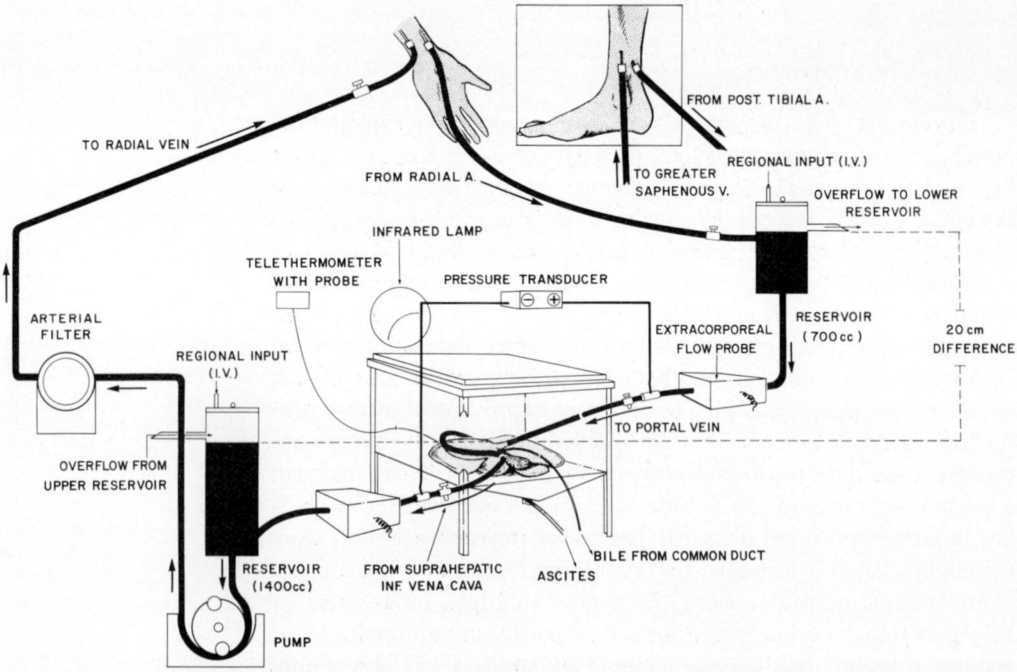

FIG. 11-3. Diagram of the perfusion system used with the *ex vivo* auxiliary pig liver. (Reproduced from McDermott, W. V., Jr., and Norman, J. C.: Metabolic Considerations in Treatment of Liver Failure With Particular Reference to Use of Ex Vivo Perfused Pig Liver. Trans. Proc. 3:1509–1517, 1971, with permission of the Publishers)

method. On the other hand, in laboratory studies, if the perfusions are widely spaced over a long time, severe anaphylactic reactions may occur, but they certainly presented no problem in closely spaced, intermittent perfusions in these severely ill patients. A number of interesting metabolic observations have been made during the course of these clinical trials and are summarized in Table 11-3.

cross circulation

Connecting the circulatory systems of a patient in acute liver failure with a volunteer with a normal liver has been tried, but the effectiveness observed has been temporary as in the *ex vivo* liver perfusion through the pig and calf liver. Hemodynamic problems may be difficult to monitor during cross circulation, and the risk of transmission of hepatitis virus is clearly considerable, although it has not

TABLE 11-3. Protein Characterization and Antibody Determinations—Results in Patients Treated with Auxiliary Pig Liver Perfusions

Protein Characterization

	Electrophoresis Pre and Post	Immunodiffusion Post		Immunoelectrophoresis Pre	Immunoelectrophoresis Post
		Human	Porcine		
Patient Sera	Atypical	Pos	Pos	Deficiency of human macroglobulins Presence of IgG (7sγ)	Presence of porcine albumin & $\alpha_{1,2}$-globulins

	Electrophoresis During	Immunodiffusion During		Immunoelectrophoresis During	
		Human	Porcine		
Porcine Liver "Ascites"	Similar to human serum pattern	Pos	Pos	Similar to human serum pattern	Porcine albumin & $\alpha_{1,2}$-globulins
Porcine Liver Bile	Presence of albumin; α,β,γ-globulins	Pos	Neg	Human serum components	Neg

Serial Antibody Determinations

	Ring	Quantitative Immuno PPT.	Immunodiffusion	Tanned RBC's
Control monospecific anti-porcine serum	Pos	Pos	Pos	Pos
All Patients	Neg	Neg	Neg	Neg

been observed in the few clinical trials to date. An ingenious technique, avoiding the problems of human volunteers, has been described independently by Hume and later by Terblanche and has been used in scattered instances elsewhere. This consists of exsanguinating a baboon under deep hypothermia, refilling his vascular system with blood that is compatible with the blood of the patient in acute liver failure and cross-perfusing baboon and patient. Technically, many of these efforts have been successful, but again, the same problems arise as have been described above with the organ perfusion techniques. In addition, careful matching for ABO compatibility must be carried out between the baboon and man.

exchange transfusion

This has been the most widely used and probably the most satisfactory of the various methods of controlling the severe metabolic derangements of a patient in fulminant hepatic failure. It certainly has the virtue of simplicity: the simultaneous withdrawal of blood from the patient and replacement with compatible donor blood is carried out using anywhere from 8 to 12 pints of donor blood. In general, because of the mixing problem it is mathematically relatively valueless to exchange more than this because, after eight replacement transfusions, it is primarily donor blood that is being withdrawn. The ease of this technique lends itself to repeated procedures at relatively short intervals. A number of patients have completely recovered after several exchange transfusions, but it is hard to compare this with other more complicated procedures of auxiliary support because one is much more inclined to use the safe and simple procedure freely whereas the more complicated and potentially more dangerous techniques have been employed only in cases in which the liver failure is clearly terminal. Nonetheless, the frequency of temporary improvement and the occasional, gratifying, long term recovery make this the procedure of choice at the moment in the management of severe and unresponsive hepatic failure.

bibliography

orthotopic liver transplantation

ACS/NIH Organ Transplant Registry: First scientific report. J. A. M. A., *217:*1520–1529, 1971.

ACS/NIH Organ Transplant Registry: Second scientific report. J. A. M. A., *221:*1486–1491, 1972.

Aune, S., Schistad, G., and Skulberg, A.: Human liver transplantation without azathioprine. Surg. Gynec. Obstet., *135:*727–728, 1972.

Aust, J. B., and Guttmann, R. D.: Factors involved in homograft tolerance. J. A. M. A., *183:*857–858, 1963.

Belzer, F. O., Ashby, B. S., Gulyassy, P. F., and Powell, M.: Successful seventeen-hour preservation and transplantation of human-cadaver kidney. New Eng. J. Med., *278:*608-610, 1968.

Burkle, J. S., et al.: The use of frozen autologous bone marrow for the protection of lethally irradiated dogs. Surg. Gynec. Obstet., *116:*600-602, 1963.

Calne, R. Y., and Williams, R.: Liver transplantation in man—I, observations on technique and organization in five cases. Brit. Med. J., *4:*535-540, 1968.

Calne, R. Y., et al.: Liver transplantation in man—II, a report of two orthotopic liver transplants in adult recipients. Brit. Med. J., *4:*541-546, 1968.

Claman, M., Balfour, J., and Forbes, D.: Survival of homologous transplants of neonatal kidneys in dogs. Surg. Gynec. Obstet., *116:*227-231, 1963.

Couch, N. P., Curran, W. J., Hyg, S. M., and Moore, F. D.: The use of cadaver tissues in transplantation. New Eng. J. Med., *271:*691-695, 1964.

Faber, L. P., Kenwell, J. M., and Beattie, E. J., Jr.: Homologous lung transplantation. Experiences in the dog. Arch. Surg., *83:*491-495, 1961.

Fortner, J. G., Shiu, M. H., Howland, W. S., and Beattie, E. J., Jr.: The donor in human liver transplantation. Surg. Gynec. Obstet., *130:*988-994, 1970.

Fortner, J. G., et al.: Orthotopic and heterotopic liver homografts in man. Ann. Surg., *172:*23-32, 1970.

Guttmann, R. D., Carpenter, C. B., Lindquist, R. R., and Merrill, J. P.: Renal transplantation in the inbred rat. III. A study of heterologous antithymocyte sera. J. Exp. Med., *126:*1099-1126, 1967.

Hardy, J. D., et al.: Heart transplantation in man. Developmental studies and report of a case. J. A. M. A., *188:*1132-1140, 1964.

Hume, D. M., et al.: Renal homotransplantation in man in modified recipients. Ann. Surg., *158:*608-644, 1963.

Jordan, G. L., Jr., Collins, V. P., and Hettig, R. A.: A study of the late effects of total body irradiation. J. A. M. A., *183:*859-860, 1963.

Lillehei, R. C., Longerbeam, J. K., and Scott, W. R.: Whole organ grafts of the stomach. J. A. M. A., *183:*861-865, 1963.

Messini, M., Cenci, G. P., and Cucchi, G.: Immunological significance of thymus. Delayed skin reaction in thymectomised rat. Lancet, *2:*180-181, 1964.

Mieny, C. J.: Haemostasis in the pig after transplantation of stored livers. S. Afr. J. Surg., *8:*15-19, 1970.

Nigro, S. L., et al.: Dogs surviving with a reimplanted lung. Bronchospirometric and pulmonary artery pressure studies. J. A. M. A., *183:*854-856, 1963.

Raju, S., Grogan, J. B., and Hardy, J. D.: Prolonged survival of skin allografts exposed to heterologous antilymphocyte serum in vitro. J. Surg. Res., *9:*327-330, 1969.

Russell, P. S., and Monaco, A. P.: The biology of tissue transplantation. New Eng. J. Med., *271:*502-510; 553-562; 610-615; 664-671; 718-725; 776-783, 1964.

Savan, B., Mooney, C. S., and Griffen, W. O., Jr.: A useful arterial anastomosis technique in orthotopic liver homotransplantation. J. Surg. Res., *10:*63-66, 1970.

Slafsky, F., Kriek, H., and Murray, J. E.: Effect of thoracic duct fistula on canine renal homografts. J. Surg. Res., *7:*105-109, 1967.

Slapak, M., Lee, H. M., and Hume, D. M.: Transplant lung—a new syndrome. Brit. Med. J. *1:*80–84, 1968.

Slapak, M., et al.: Effect of heparin, arvin, liver perfusion, and heterologous antiplatelet serum on rejection of pig kidney by dog. Transplantation Proc., *3:*558–561, 1971.

Starzl, T. E.: Heterologous antilymphocyte globulin. New Eng. J. Med., *279:*700–703, 1968.

Starzl, T. E.: Experience in Hepatic Transplantation. Philadelphia, W. B. Saunders Co., 1969, 533 pp.

Varco, R. L., Maclean, L. D., Aust, J. B., and Good, R. A.: Agammaglobulinemia: An approach to homovital transplantation. Ann. Surg., *142:*334–344, 1955.

auxiliary liver transplantation

Giles, G., et al.: Effect of auxiliary liver transplantation on haptoglobin synthesis in the dog. Surg. Forum, *20:*367–369, 1969.

Halgrimson, C. G., et al.: Auxiliary liver transplantation: Effect of host portacaval shunt. Experimental and clinical observations. Arch. Surg., *93:*107–118, 1966.

van der Heyde, M. N., Schalm, L., and Vink, M.: The role of functional competition in auxiliary liver transplantation. Transplantation, *5:*78–80, 1967.

van der Heyde, M. N., Cooper, J. R., Carter, J. H., and Welch, C. S.: Survival of hepatectomized dogs with partial liver transplants. Surgery, *59:*1079–1082, 1967.

Kuster, G. G. R., and Woods, J. E.: Auxiliary liver transplantation in the dog as temporary support in acute fulminating hepatic necrosis. Ann. Surg., *176:*732–735, 1972.

Maki, T., Blackburn, G. L., Slapak, M., and McDermott, W. V., Jr.: A life supporting heterotopic autotransplant of the canine liver without portal blood. Surg. Gynec. Obstet. (in press).

Malt, R. A., et al.: Auxiliary partial liver transplantation in *Macaca mulatta.* Ann. Surg., *171:*575–582, 1970.

Marchioro, T. L., et al.: Physiologic requirements for auxiliary liver homotransplantation. Surg. Gynec. Obstet., *121:*17–31, 1965.

Melin, M., et al.: 'Haptoglobin' after liver transplantation in dogs. Vox Sang., *17:*74–75, 1969.

Mito, M., et al.: Partial heterotopic liver homograft in dogs utilizing portal arterialization. Ann. Surg., *165:*20–32, 1967.

Ranson, J. H. C., Garcia-Moran, M., Becker, F. F., and Localio, S. A.: Portal inflow and auxiliary hepatic allograft function. Surg. Gynec. Obstet., *135:*769–776, 1972.

Slapak, M., Beaudoin, J. G., Lee, H. M., and Hume, D. M.: Auxiliary liver homotransplantation. A new technique and an evaluation of current techniques. Arch. Surg., *100:*31–41, 1970.

Tamvakopoulos, S. K., and Randall, H. T.: One year survival and function after heterotopic liver autotransplantation. Surg. Gynec. Obstet., *130:* 859–864, 1970.

Wexler, M. J., et al.: Auxiliary liver transplantation: A successful model without portal blood or portacaval shunt. Ann. Surg., *175:*357–374, 1972.

liver preservation

Slapak, M., Wigmore, R. A., and MacLean, L. D.: Twenty-four hour liver preservation by the use of continuous pulsatile perfusion and hyperbaric oxygen. Transplantation, *5:*1154–1158, 1967.

Slapak, M., et al.: Organ preservation using a simple portable apparatus suitable for controlled hyperbaric conditions. *In* Norman, J. C., et al. (Eds.): Organ Perfusion and Preservation. New York, Appleton-Century-Crofts, 1968, pp. 317–335.

Slapak, M., et al.: Asanguinous perfusion preservation of canine liver and heart using a simple manuable portable apparatus. Transplantation Proc., *1:*147–152, 1969.

Slapak, M., et al.: Extended preservation of the primate liver by simple cooling and orthotopic auto transplantation. Surg. Forum, *21:*348–350, 1970.

Spilg, H., et al.: Successful liver transplantation after storage for 6–8 hours, using a simple hypothermic immersion technique. Transplantation, *11:*457–460, 1971.

Wexler, M., et al.: Regeneration and maintenance of integrity of canine liver. The role of arterial, portal, and systemic venous blood. Arch. Surg., *101:*267–276, 1970.

Willman, V. L., Cooper, T., Cian, L. G., and Hanlon, C. R.: Autotransplantation of the canine heart. Surg. Gynec. Obstet., *115:*299–302, 1962.

auxiliary liver perfusion

Battersby, C., Winch, J., Balderson, G., and Burnett, W.: Immunological results of hepatic assistance procedures. J. Surg. Res., *11:*179–186, 1971.

Cuschieri, A., Baker, P. R., and Shields, R.: Auxiliary liver perfusion in the pig. Effect of ischaemically damaged livers on recipient animals. J. Surg. Res., *13:*188–196, 1972.

Drapanas, T., Semel, R., and Vang, J. O.: Hemodynamics of the isolated perfused pig liver: Metabolism according to routes of perfusion and rates of flow. Ann. Surg., *164:*522–537, 1966.

Eiseman, B.: Treatment of hepatic coma by extracorporeal liver perfusion. Ann. Roy. Coll. Surg. Eng., *38:*329–348, 1966.

Eiseman, B., Liem, D. S., and Raffucci, F.: Heterologous liver perfusion in treatment of hepatic failure. Ann. Surg., *162:*329–345, 1965.

Hardison, W. G. M., Greene, E. A., and Norman, J. C.: The viability and effect of flow upon function of the ex vivo perfused pig liver. J. Lab. Clin. Med., *69:*245–255, 1967.

Norman, J. C., Hardison, W. G., and McDermott, W. V., Jr.: Therapeutic and investigational potential of heterologous liver perfusion. Bull. N.Y. Acad. Med., *43:*967–976, 1967.

Norman, J. C., Brown, M., Ackroyd, F. W., and McDermott, W. V., Jr.: Effect of increasing outflow occlusion on the rate and composition of ascites formation by the isolated perfused porcine liver. Surg. Forum, *16:*276–278, 1965.

Norman, J. C., et al.: Perfusion techniques in temporary human-isolated ex vivo porcine liver cross circulation. Possible adjunct in the treatment of hepatic failure. J. Surg. Res., *6:*121–125, 1966.

Norman, J. C., et al.: Techniques of obtaining and preparing the porcine liver for experimental and clinical ex vivo perfusion. J. Surg. Res., *6:*117–120, 1966.

Tait, I. B., and Eiseman, B.: Perfusion dynamics for extracorporeal hepatic assist. Arch. Surg., *93:*131–141, 1966.

exchange transfusion

Abouna, G. M.: Improved technique of exchange transfusion for hepatic coma. Surg. Gynec. Obstet., *134:*658–662, 1972.

Barlyn, L. E., Trey, C., Fagan, J. F., and McDermott, W. V., Jr.: Exchange transfusion for fulminant hepatic failure following hepatic resection. Arch. Surg., *102:*224–226, 1971.

Berger, R. L., et al.: Exchange transfusion in the treatment of fulminating hepatitis. New Eng. J. Med., *274:*497–499, 1966.

Klebanoff, G., et al.: Resuscitation of a patient in stage IV hepatic coma using total body washout. J. Surg. Res., *13:*159–165, 1972.

Klebanoff, G., et al.: Asanguineous hypothermic total body perfusion (TBW) in the treatment of stage IV hepatic coma. J. Surg. Res., *12:*1–7, 1972.

Krebs, R., and Flynn, M.: Treatment of hepatic coma with exchange transfusion and peritoneal dialysis. J. A. M. A., *198:*430–432, 1967.

Lee, C., and Tink, A.: Exchange transfusion in hepatic coma: Report of a case. Med. J. Aust., *1:*40–42, 1958.

Trey, C., Burns, D. G., and Saunders, S. J.: Treatment of hepatic coma by exchange blood transfusion. New Eng. J. Med., *274:*473–481, 1966.

Trey, C., et al.: Massive liver necrosis in the monkey: The effects of exchange blood transfusions on fulminant liver failure. J. Lab. Clin. Med., *73:*784–794, 1969.

hemodialysis and peritoneal dialysis

Keynes, W. M.: Hemodialysis of ammonium nitrogen. Surg. Gynec. Obstet., *132:*657–661, 1971.

Kiley, J. E., Pender, J. C., Welch, H. F., and Welch, C. S.: Ammonia intoxication treated by hemodialysis. New Eng. J. Med., *259:*1156–1161, 1958.

Kiley, J. E., Welch, H. F., Pender, J. C., and Welch, C. S.: Removal of blood ammonia by hemodialysis. Proc. Soc. Exp. Biol. Med., *91:*489–493, 1956.

Ritchie, H. D., et al.: Extracorporeal methods of reducing high blood ammonia levels. Gut, *3:*172–176, 1962.

cross circulation

Burnell, J. M., et al.: Acute hepatic coma treated by cross-circulation or exchange transfusion. New Eng. J. Med., *276:*935–943, 1967.

Joyeuse, R., Ivanisevic, B., Longmire, W. P., Jr., and Maloney, J. V., Jr.: The treatment of experimental hepatic coma by parabiotic cross circulation. Surg. Gynec. Obstet., *117:*129–138, 1963.

Nienhuis, L. I., Mulmed, E. I., and Kelly, J. W.: Hepatic coma. Treatment emphasizing merit of peritoneal dialysis. Amer. J. Surg., *106:*980–985, 1963.

Saunders, S. J., Bosman, S. C. W., Bernard, C. N., and Terblanche, J.: The use of exchange transfusions and cross-circulation with the baboon in the treatment of fulminant liver failure. Present Concepts, *2:*161–180, 1969.

Storb, R., et al.: Clinical and hematologic effects of cross circulation in baboons. Transfusion, *9:*23–31, 1969.

Trauma of the Liver

CHAPTER 12

Surgical references to hepatic trauma tend, of necessity, to be anecdotal in character; it is extremely difficult to set up a specific classification because of the tremendous variety in the types of missiles or instruments causing damage to the liver, the increasing incidence of blunt trauma with varying degrees of severity of impact and the occurrence of injuries to extrahepatic related structures and other organs that complicate surgical repair and alter mortality. It is, thus, not easy to derive comparable mortality figures because every reported series tends to be weighted with variations in the nature of the severity of the damage incurred. We do not intend to present a comprehensive survey of all the reported experience in the number of wars that have occurred in this century or the extensive experience available on civilian injuries both from penetrating and from blunt trauma. Obviously, the availability of early surgical attention is a major factor influencing mortality, and therefore the results of varying approaches to liver injury and differences in military and civilian experience are difficult to analyze.

Matting and Kennedy have written an excellent monograph on liver trauma in which all the important aspects of the problem have been defined and discussed in considerable detail. In this chapter we will not attempt to be all inclusive, but rather we will attempt to present a classification of liver injury that is not so much anatomic as descriptive of the severity of the damage and the attendant degree of complexity of the surgery involved.

classification

In Table 12-1, we have attempted to present a classification of liver injury that may be useful in categorizing a subject of tremendous variability into compartments that relate to the extensiveness of the damage and, therefore, the complexity of the surgery rather than to

TABLE 12-1. Classification of Liver Trauma

A. Penetrating or perforating wounds
   1. Low velocity instrument
      a. Without associated injury
      b. With associated injury
   2. High velocity missile
      a. Without associated injury
      b. With associated injury
B. Blunt trauma

any anatomic definition. In Figure 12-1A to 12-1E a pictorial view of the classification is presented with examples of the types of surgery that might be applicable to these particular situations.

Penetrating or *perforating wounds* of the liver may, of course, involve any combination of the anatomic segments of the liver. Since the right lobe of the liver comprises approximately 85 per cent of its total mass, it is obviously the most common location for this type of injury, although obviously any missile or instrument can inflict a wound that involves all the anatomic segments. The extensiveness of the injury, the complexity of the surgery and the ultimate mortality probably relate more to the velocity of the missile or instrument inflicting the injury and the presence or absence of adjacent damage than to any other factors.

In the case of low velocity bullets, metal fragments or instruments such as knives and ice picks, evaluation of the tract will give some initial indication of the amount of damage incurred. In low velocity injury, there is relatively little spreading force so that one would not anticipate extensive parenchymal damage much beyond the actual tract itself. It is this type of injury that often can be handled by exploration of the wounds of entrance and of exit (if present), temporary packing to control bleeding and then individual ligation of transected vascular and biliary channels. If the injury is peripheral in either the right or left lobe, a limited resection and mattress suture closure may be the most effective and expeditious method of management. Packing with gauze or with hemostatic materials is to be avoided unless this proves to be the only possible way of controlling a potentially lethal hemorrhage.

In the case of high velocity missiles, a different situation frequently exists. Even though the wounds of entrance and exit may seem of relatively negligible consequence, there is often an extensive area of intrahepatic damage as a result of the passage of the missile through the liver. This is very difficult to evaluate, but if the operating surgeon explores the wound of entrance or exit with his finger, he may find that the tract has a firm, resilient wall in the case of a low velocity missile. If extensive intrahepatic damage has occurred, he may find

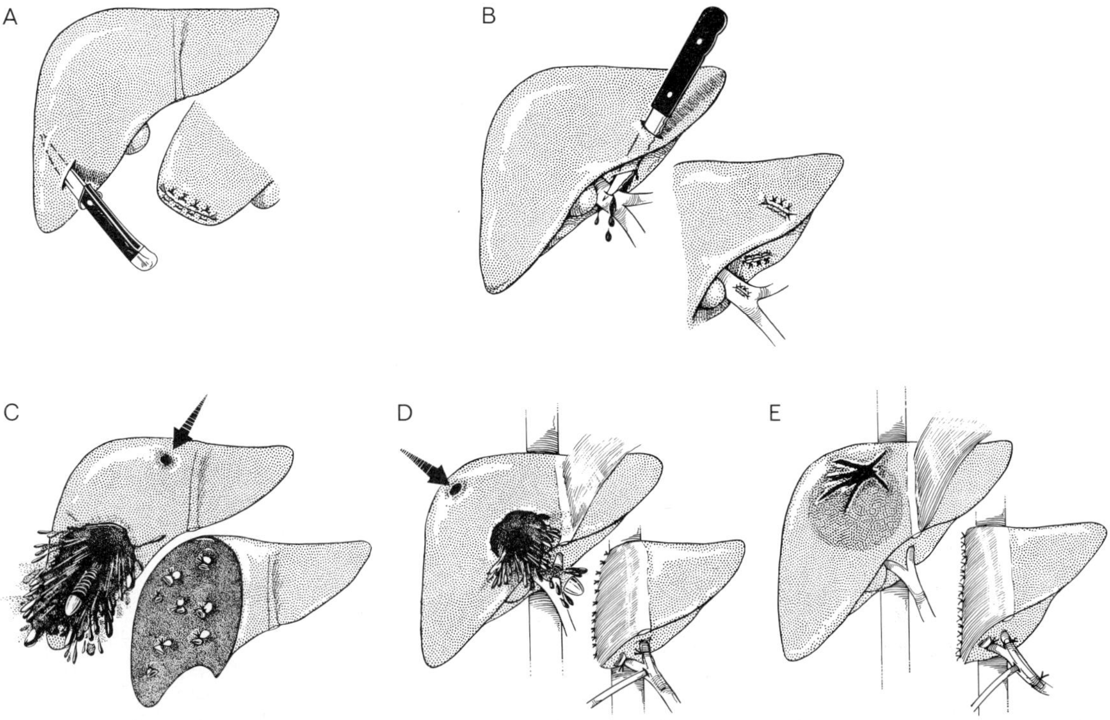

FIG. 12-1. A, Penetrating wound (low velocity instrument) without associated injury. B, Penetrating wound (low velocity instrument) with associated injury. C, Penetrating wound (high velocity missile) without associated injury. D, Penetrating wound (high velocity missile) with associated injury. E, Blunt trauma

that his exploring finger drops into a rather gelatinous mass of destroyed liver parenchyma. Sometimes the presence of bits of liver tissue extruded from the injury into the abdominal cavity may give the clue to the presence of a more extensive injury than had been initially expected.

If extrahepatic injury occurs, the problem clearly becomes more complicated. With the entrance of any missile or instrument into the abdominal cavity, injury may occur to a number of different organs. It is beyond the scope of this particular review to consider all the possible combinations of injuries that may occur within the peritoneal or retroperitoneal areas, so comments will be limited to the immediate extrahepatic structures. When the injury in any way approaches the anatomic hilus of the liver, one must carefully inspect the structures of the gastrohepatic ligament, since occult injuries to the extrahepatic biliary tract, hepatic artery or portal vein may be present and then result in lethal complications if corrective surgery is not applied at the time of the initial operation. If the tract of the injury raises the suspicion of penetration posteriorly, the right lobe of the liver should be mobilized so the area of the hepatic veins and the vena cava can be inspected. Sometimes hemorrhage from injury to these vessels may be arrested temporarily because of hypotension and transient occlusion by clots. This type of situation may lead to disastrous postoperative hemorrhage, and it is important to assure the integrity of these vessels at the time of the initial exploration. Injuries to the hepatic vein or vena cava are, in fact, the cause of the majority of the fatal outcomes encountered in liver injuries. Hemorrhage may be massive and almost uncontrollable. A number of suggestions have been made such as the introduction of balloons into the vena cava, the isolation of the vena cava within the pericardium and a number of other technical innovations relating to specific instruments designed or employed towards this purpose. In fact, the situations encountered require individual solutions and therefore are dependent on the imagination and versatility of the surgeon. The principles, however, are clear. Immediate inflow occlusion can be obtained with any relatively nontraumatic temporary occluding clamp. Rapid isolation of the vena cava above and below the liver with temporary occluding tapes will then permit a somewhat more leisurely exploration of the injury and ligation or repair of the vessels injured.

Occlusion of the inflow to the liver presents two major problems: One relates to the safe time of total ischemia, and the second, to the fact that outflow from the splanchnic bed is obstructed, and therefore recompartmentalization of the available blood volume occurs with pooling in that area and relative hypovolemia elsewhere. Recognition of the pooling phenomenon requires additional transfusion beyond what would be required by the actual measured blood loss.

Problems relating to ischemia of the liver have been the source of innumerable clinical and experimental reports. The safe ischemia time of the normothermic liver has been given as ranging from 20 minutes to one hour. Hypothermia obviously increases the safe period of hepatic ischemia, and many authors have suggested that this is a valuable adjunct to surgery of the liver. Our own feeling is that this would be rarely, if ever, a useful maneuver regardless of the mechanism by which hypothermia is induced. Any method for significant lowering of hepatic temperature requires a certain amount of time, and the occasions when it might be useful are so catastrophic that immediate rather than delayed surgical action is required. There is certainly no objection to cooling by use of a blanket during vigorous efforts at controlling hemorrhage, but in most circumstances either the hemorrhage will be controlled before effective hypothermia has been induced or the patient will have died from exsanguination and cardiac arrest.

Blunt trauma occurs with increasing frequency as the volume of high speed traffic on large highways increases. Frequently this presents more difficult diagnostic problems than does penetrating trauma because there may be little or no external evidence to point to injury occurring in the area of the right upper quadrant. Even when exploration is clearly indicated, the location and extent of injury to the liver may be surprisingly obscure. In this type of implosion injury, the only external evidence on the liver may be the presence of a relatively innocuous looking stellate laceration on the dome of the right lobe beneath the diaphragm (Fig. 12-1E). Unless the right lobe is mobilized and this area inspected carefully, the injury is not easily visible. Even when it is visualized, there may be a temptation to occlude the obvious injury with mattress sutures, and this, in fact, may result in temporary cessation of bleeding. Most of these injuries, however, involve extensive intrahepatic damage with reduction of a significant portion of the liver tissue to a pulpy mass. In this instance in particular, the type of finger exploration referred to above is especially valuable and may be the only thing that will point to the necessity of a major hepatic resection with removal of the devitalized tissue rather than temporary occlusion of the external injury with mattress sutures.

occlusion of hepatic blood supply

The exigencies involved in the control of traumatic hemorrhage from the liver may raise the question of ligation of either the hepatic artery or portal vein, as may the existence of irreparable injury to either. It is important, therefore, to analyze the effects of varying degrees of inflow occlusion to the liver. Ligation of *both* the proper hepatic and the main portal veins is invariably fatal. Beyond this, there is considerable variation in clinical and experimental preparations.

Occlusion of the *portal vein* without establishment of some type of portal-systemic shunt was considered for many years to be lethal. It is true that ligation of the superior mesenteric or portal vein in the dog results in death within a few hours, but Child, using the *Macaca mulatta* monkey as an experimental animal, showed that survival was the rule rather than the exception and that this was because of the existence of a much richer portal-systemic collateral system than occurs in the dog and other animals. Extending these observations further, Child ligated the portal vein with no adverse effects in several patients with terminal malignant disease. He then felt it justifiable to resect the portal vein in patients with invasive carcinoma of the head of the pancreas in a two stage procedure in which the portal vein was ligated initially. Within a few weeks, the immediate portal hypertension had subsided and pancreaticoduodenectomy could be carried out successfully. Many subsequent observations by ourselves and others have confirmed the fact that, in man, permanent occlusion of the portal vein results in immediate portal hypertension, sequestration of a significant portion of the blood volume in the splanchnic bed and a decrease in blood volume. These effects are transient, however, and disappear as natural portal-systemic shunts open up.

Since *ligation of the hepatic artery* has been suggested and utilized as a means of controlling hemorrhage from an injured liver, it is important to understand the results of occlusion at varying points in the arterial inflow.

The portal venous inflow represents, under normal conditions, about 80 per cent of the total hepatic blood flow. Portal blood has a higher oxygen saturation than peripheral venous blood. Therefore, one might anticipate that viability of the liver could be maintained by the portal circulation alone; in fact, this appears to be true in most cases. Certainly, ligation of the hepatic artery proximal to the gastroduodenal artery has no demonstrable effect on liver function or viability. Distal to this point, however, ligation of the proper hepatic artery or one of its major branches has variable effects, depending on the collateral circulation available and on the clinical condition of the patient. In shock, the portal flow is significantly decreased, and interruption of the major arterial supply can result in diffuse hepatic necrosis and death.

On the other hand, there are numerous case reports in the literature indicating that permanent occlusion of the proper hepatic artery or one of the major branches is quite compatible with survival. Ligation of the right or left hepatic artery has been used in the management of malignant disease of the liver to induce regression of tumor prior to resection. In cirrhosis, multiple arterial ligations in the celiac circulation had been used to decrease inflow and reduce portal hypertension; some favorable results were achieved but the overall mortality was high and hepatic necrosis frequent. Better understanding of the hemodynamics of portal hypertension makes these discrepancies understandable. In early cirrhosis, portal flow to the liver is nearly normal; with progressive fibrosis and increasing postsinusoidal block, portal flow decreases and blood supply is maintained by a compensatory increase in arterial flow. Under these circumstances, interruption of the artery may be and has been followed by fatal hepatic necrosis.

Beyond determining the mortality after arterial ligations at various points in the circulation, effects under clinical conditions are difficult to analyze. In our own experience, ligation of a major arterial branch may be attended by partial atrophy of the area supplied. Two brief case reports are illustrative:

CASE 1. A 79 year old man was admitted with painless obstructive jaundice. A mass was palpable in the epigastrium, interpreted as metastatic disease. Ten years before, a cholecystectomy had been carried out elsewhere and had been attended by a prolonged convalescence with high fever. At exploration, a "silent" common duct stone was found to be the cause of the biliary obstruction. The right lobe of the liver was fibrotic and atrophied, and the left lobe was hypertrophied, forming the epigastric mass described on physical examination. Dissection of the gastrohepatic ligament demonstrated that the right hepatic artery had been inadvertently ligated at the time of the previous cholecystectomy.

CASE 2. A 36 year old woman was admitted for repair of a stricture of the extrahepatic biliary tract from an injury sustained at elective cholecystectomy four months previously. Convalescence had been predictably complicated with fever and profuse drainage. At the time of repair of the damaged common hepatic duct, the right lobe of the liver was atrophic and the left hypertrophied. Dissection prior to excision and repair of the stricture revealed that the right hepatic artery was involved in the scar of the stricture and had been completely occluded.

Summarizing the rather sparse information available, one could presume that (1) ligation of the proximal common hepatic artery does not appreciably interfere with hepatic blood flow; (2) ligation of the proper hepatic artery (distal to the gastroduodenal artery) is usually not fatal unless portal blood flow is significantly decreased by shock; (3) ligation of the right or left hepatic artery may be followed by atrophy of the supplied lobe and compensatory hypertrophy of the other. Therefore, there is a considerable margin of safety if circumstances attendant upon liver injury require some type of arterial ligation to control exsanguinating hemorrhage.

Most of the *late mortality* in hepatic trauma occurs because of failure to employ major hepatic resection and remove extensively devitalized hepatic parenchyma. Two case histories cited below represent vivid examples of delayed complications that were nearly fatal as well as of instances in which major hepatic resection would have been advisable at the initial operation.

CASE 3. The patient, a 47 year old man, suffered severe blunt abdominal trauma in an automobile accident four weeks prior to admission. Severe, deep liver lacerations were produced and were treated elsewhere with suture of the hepatic capsule. Ten days prior to the patient's transfer, the course became septic; referral for emergency management was necessitated by massive hemorrhage and septicemia. Angiography demonstrated a large intrahepatic abscess with multiple arteriovenous fistulas (Fig. 12-2). The patient underwent an emergency right hepatic lobectomy through a thoracoabdominal incision with insertion of a common duct T-tube and appropriate drains. The postoperative course was complicated by a lung abscess in the right lower lobe and homologous serum jaundice, both of which eventually cleared with conservative management over a three month period. He is now alive and in good health.

Comment. The case illustrates the complications of recurrent hemorrhage and sepsis, which may attend suture and packing in extensive liver injury, and points up the importance of anatomic resection when indicated by the extent of devitalized tissue.

CASE 4. The patient, an 18 year old girl, suffered blunt abdominal trauma in an automobile accident and was admitted to the accident room in shock. Exploratory laparotomy revealed a deep laceration of the dome of the right lobe of the liver; this was initially packed, drains were placed and the abdomen closed. Two hours after the exploration, the abdomen became distended and the patient became hypotensive;

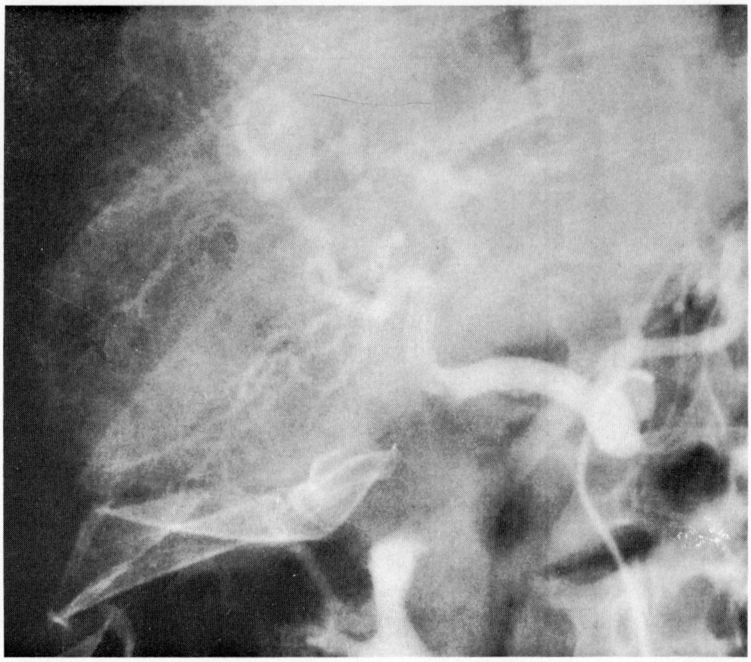

FIG. 12-2. Selective hepatic arteriogram (Case 3) showing post-traumatic hepatic abscess

it became apparent that intraperitoneal hemorrhage had recurred. The abdomen was re-explored, and right hepatic lobectomy was carried out through a thoracoabdominal approach. The patient tolerated the procedure well, requiring a total of 13 units of blood. A T-tube was placed in the common duct and sump drains were placed in the operative area. Pleural effusions developed on the right side; they were tapped and proved to be sterile. Pneumothorax involving 20 per cent of the right side was noted, but re-expansion gradually occurred. The patient was discharged in good condition one month after hepatic resection.

Comment. The rapid recurrence of massive hemorrhage after mattress suture control emphasizes the role of emergency resection as an initial procedure in selected cases of liver trauma.

clinical approach to liver injury

With the background of the general concepts outlined above, one can then begin to define a general approach to hepatic trauma. Suspicion of the injury is obviously of vital importance since this should lead progressively to accurate diagnosis and early operation. In the majority of cases, the surgeon will be confronted with the necessity of immediate laparotomy because of continued severe intra-abdominal hemorrhage often defined by the use of peritoneal tap. If liver injury is suspected and the patient's condition is sufficiently stable, there may be instances in which the use of selected celiac arteriography may be extremely helpful. This can be done quickly, and certainly is extremely helpful in indicating the extent of the intrahepatic injury, which, as stated above, may not be easily apparent at exploration. When this procedure is neither feasible nor safe, early operation with a right upper quadrant paramedian incision is indicated. The extent of damage to the liver can be initially evaluated through this approach. Sometimes the operative procedure required, whether peripheral resection or suture ligation and closure, can be accomplished without further extension of the incision. The patient should, however, be positioned and prepared in such a way that extension of the abdominal incision through the bed of the 5th or 6th rib or in the appropriate interspace is possible. This extension is frequently required when major hepatic lobectomy is indicated, when the injury occurs at the dome or posterior part of the liver or when retrohepatic vessels are the source of continued hemorrhage. Following the principles outlined above, the surgeon reaches his decision as to the type of reparative surgery required (either ligation and closure or resection of varying extent). Having assured himself that no extrahepatic injury has occurred or having corrected any of the vascular or biliary injuries that have resulted from the trauma, the surgeon may then close the incision with appropriate drainage in which some suction should be utilized if any significant bile leakage is expected. Choledochotomy and T-tube drainage have been discussed extensively in surgical circles, and it is our opinion that this is extremely valuable unless the common bile duct is unusually small and, therefore, subject to a significant risk of late stricture. The placement of a T-tube in the common duct has a number of advantages. Firstly, prior to closure, the T-tube may be irrigated under gentle pressure with colored saline. The appearance of this colored solution at any point on the cut surface of the liver may be the only indication of an open bile duct, which could result in prolonged biliary fistula unless occluded with a ligature at the time of the initial operation. Secondly, it also permits evaluation of the nature and volume of the bile flow in the postoperative period. Hemobilia is not an uncommon sequel to extensive liver injury; unless by utilization of the presence of a T-tube the source of the bleeding can be immediately pointed out, it may present only as gastrointestinal bleeding and other sources be suspected rather than the true origin within the liver. Thirdly, an intrahepatic area of hematoma or devitalized tissue may exist without recognition at the initial procedure and with delayed infection may be the source of unexplained fever and sepsis postoperatively. Cholangiography through the T-tube may define this source of otherwise unexplained sepsis and will also serve to locate the origin of a persistent bile leak.

major hepatic resection

Elsewhere in this book, both the technique of major hepatic resection and the metabolic problems encountered postoperatively have been discussed in detail and need not be repeated here. Suffice it to say that the average general surgeon is not likely to encounter many cases in which elective right hepatic lobectomy is required, but inevitably he will encounter cases of severe hepatic trauma in which this is the procedure of choice. When the established principle of removal of devitalized and seriously damaged hepatic parenchyma is followed, the removal of the right lobe and the medial segment of the left lobe along with the caudate and quadrate lobes is not infrequently indicated and lifesaving. If the injury extends into the left lobe and the medial segment of this is included in the resection, the surgeon should have a probe introduced through a choledochotomy into the left hepatic bile duct since this may lie very close to the resection margin and is easily damaged permanently at the time of the rapid resection. The metabolic problems in the postoperative period have been defined in detail elsewhere and may be summarized by emphasizing the necessity of continuous glucose infusions during the first 48 hours, acceptance of a low bile flow and some degree of bilirubinemia and the requirement for parenteral administration of human serum albumin in amounts adequate to maintain a normal level and satisfactory intravascular osmotic pressure.

postoperative abscess

The occurrence of subhepatic and subphrenic abscesses subsequent to operation for hepatic trauma is all too frequent. If attention is paid to the principle of removal of all devitalized liver tissue at the initial operation, the frequency of these abscesses should decrease significantly. They are often difficult to locate, and accurate identification by scintiscan arteriography, fluoroscopy and other radiographic techniques will provide the clue to the appropriate incision and drainage.

hemobilia

While this is not a frequent sequel to hepatic injury, it does occur and presents considerable difficulty in management. Sandblom and Sparkman have both reported series of post-traumatic hemobilia, frequently following nonpenetrating injuries to the liver with unrecognized extensive intrahepatic parenchymal damage. The presence of a T-tube in the common duct is of great advantage in early diagnosis and frequently in delineation of the area of the liver that is the source of the bleeding. Selective hepatic arteriography frequently demonstrates a blush at the point of an arterial biliary communication and thus points to the appropriate operative procedure for control. If a T-tube is not present and if arteriography is not helpful, scintiscan using ^{131}I-labeled rose bengal or colloidal gold (^{198}Au) may be very helpful. More recently, technetium sulfur colloid has been used preferentially by many radiologists.

The treatment of hemobilia depends on the location and the nature of the source. If the vascular biliary fistula is peripheral or is near the surface of the central portion of the liver, exteriorization and drainage with ligation of the injured vessels may be sufficient. Frequently the lesion is deep in liver substance, and formal hepatic resection may be required once localization has been achieved.

bile peritonitis

It is surprising that with the extensive literature available on this subject there is so little agreement among surgeons today. Some of the confusion at least results from the differing composition of bile in experimental animals and the varying toxicity of the different bile salts. Certainly bilirubin itself is nontoxic, and human bile salts are less toxic than those occurring in many animals. Under clinical circumstances the free entrance of bile into the abdominal cavity is so often accompanied by other serious problems that the pathophysiologic effects of the bile alone are difficult to evaluate. Bile salts are unquestionably irritating, and chemical peritonitis does occur, but whether this of itself can be lethal is doubtful. Some loss of fluids and electrolytes and a depletion in plasma volume may occur, but adequate replacement should control this aspect of the problem. It has been suggested but never satisfactorily established that the chemical effects of bile render the area more susceptible to invasive or localized infection. Regardless of the absolute facts, few surgeons would disagree with the dogma that actual or potential bile leakage should be managed by drainage adequate to establish an external biliary fistula.

summary

While injuries to the liver are extremely varied and individual considerations are important in management, certain generalizations are useful and basic principles are applicable.

1. The extent of penetrating or perforating injury is dependent both on the nature of the missile or instrument and on the anatomic tract. Resection is more frequently indicated when the injury is caused by a high velocity missile causing extensive damage beyond the tract itself.

2. The devitalization of hepatic parenchyma by blunt trauma is often more extensive than would appear from casual inspection. Failure to resect necrotic tissue will result in serious and often fatal complications (intrahepatic abscess, hemobilia, septicemia, delayed intra-abdominal hemorrhage, etc.).

3. If circumstances permit, selective hepatic arteriography is valuable in identifying the extent of the injury.

4. Hypothermia has not, in our experience, been a useful adjunct to the management of liver injury.

bibliography

Ackroyd, F. W., Pollard, J., and McDermott, W. V., Jr.: Massive hepatic resection in the treatment of severe liver trauma. Amer. J. Surg., *117:* 442–448, 1969.

Albo, D., Jr., Christensen, C., Rasmussen, B. L., and King, T. C.: Massive liver trauma involving the suprarenal vena cava. Amer. J. Surg., *118:* 960–963, 1969.

Aronsen, K. F., et al.: Liver resection in the treatment of blunt injuries to the liver. Surgery, *63:*236–246, 1968.

Brittain, R. S.: Liver trauma. Surg. Clin. N. Amer., *43:*433–444, 1963.

Brittain, R. S., et al.: Accidental hepatic artery ligation in humans. Amer. J. Surg., *107:*822–832, 1964.

Byrne, R. V.: The surgical repair of major liver injuries. Surg. Gynec. Obstet., *119:*113–115, 1964.

Child, C. G., III: The Liver and Portal Hypertension. Philadelphia, W. B. Saunders Co., 1964, 231 pp.

Child, C. G., III, Milnes, R. F., Holswade, G. R., and Gore, A. L.: Sudden and complete occlusion of the portal vein in the *Macaca mulatta* monkey. Ann. Surg., *132:*475–495, 1950.

Cohn, I., Jr., et al.: Bile peritonitis. Ann. Surg., *152:*827–835, 1960.

Graff, R. J.: Considerations in the treatment of traumatic hemobilia. Amer. J. Surg., *105:*662–666, 1963.

Graham, W. P., III, Eiseman, B., and Pryor, R.: Hepatic artery aneurysm with portal vein fistula in a patient with familial hereditary telangiectasia. Ann. Surg., *159:*362–367, 1964.

Hardy, K. J.: Patterns of liver injury after fatal blunt trauma. Surg. Gynec. Obstet., *134:*39–43, 1972.

Hendren, W. H., Warshaw, A. L., Fleischli, D. J., and Bartlett, M. K.: Traumatic hemobilia: Non-operative management with healing documented by serial angiography. Ann. Surg., *174:*991–993, 1971.

Hermann, R. E., and Hoerr, S. O.: Aids in the diagnosis of traumatic hemobilia. Surg. Gynec. Obstet., *125:*55–58, 1967.

Horrall, O. H.: The toxicity of bile. Physiol. Rev., *11:*122–142, 1931.

Inui, F. K., and Ferguson, T. A.: Aneurysm of the right hepatic artery. Preoperative diagnosis and successful excision. Ann. Surg., *144:*235–239, 1956.

Jordan, P. H., Jr.: Treatment of amebic abscess of the liver by open surgical drainage. Ann. Surg., *141:*70–76, 1955.

Judd, D. R., and Moore T. C.: Right hepatic lobectomy for massive liver trauma: Case report. Ann. Surg., *163:*149–152, 1966.

Karasewich, E. G., and Bowden, L.: Hepatic artery injury. Surg. Gynec. Obstet., *124:*1057–1063, 1967.

Kirklin, J. W., Shocket, E., Comfort, M. W., and Huizenga, K. A.: Treatment of aneurysm of the hepatic artery by excision. Report of case. Ann. Surg., *142:*110–114, 1955.

Lucas, C. E., and Walt, A. J.: Critical decisions in liver trauma. Experience based on 604 cases. Arch. Surg., *101:*277–283, 1970.

Madding, G. F.: Injuries of the liver. Arch. Surg., *70:*748–756, 1955.

Madding, G. F., and Kennedy, P. A.: Trauma to the Liver. 2nd Ed. Philadelphia, W. B. Saunders Co., 1971, 186 pp.

Madding, G. F., and Peniston, W. H.: Collective review. Liver hemostasis. Int. Abstr. Surg., *104:*417–424, 1957.

Madding, G. F., Kennedy, P. A., and Sogemeier, E.: Hepatic artery ligation for metastatic tumor in the liver. Amer. J. Surg., *120:*95-96, 1970.

Mays, E. T.: Observations and management after hepatic artery ligation. Surg. Gynec. Obstet., *124:*801-807, 1967.

Mays, E. T.: Complex penetrating hepatic wounds. Ann. Surg., *173:*421-428, 1971.

McClelland, R., Shires, T., and Poulos, E.: Hepatic resection for massive trauma. J. Trauma, *4:*282-291, 1964.

McDermott, W. V., Jr., Greenberger, M. J., Isselbacher, K. J., and Weber, A. L.: Major hepatic resection: Diagnostic techniques and metabolic problems. Surgery, *54:*56-66, 1963.

Merendino, K. A., Dillard, D. H., and Cammock, E. E.: The concept of surgical biliary decompression in the management of liver trauma. Surg. Gynec. Obstet., *117:*285-293, 1963.

Miller, E. M.: Abdominal injuries due to blunt force. Surg. Gynec. Obstet., *106:*355-357, 1958.

Payne, W. D., Terz, J. J., and Lawrence, W., Jr.: Major hepatic resection for trauma. Ann. Surg., *170:*929-936, 1969.

Pilcher, D. B.: Penetrating injuries of the liver in Vietnam. Ann. Surg., *170:*793-800, 1969.

Poulos, E.: Hepatic resection for massive liver injuries. Ann. Surg., *157:* 525-531, 1963.

Quattlebaum, J. K.: Aneurysm of the hepatic artery: Report of three cases. Ann. Surg., *139:*743-750, 1954.

Shackelford, R. T., and Marbury, W. B., Jr.: Left hepatic lobectomy for external biliary fistula. Ann. Surg., *144:*245-251, 1956.

Souliotis, P. T., Pettigrew, A. H., and Chamberlain, J. W.: Traumatic hemobilia. New Eng. J. Med., *268:*565-568, 1963.

Sparkman, R. S., and Fogelman, M. J.: Wounds of the liver. Review of 100 cases. Ann. Surg., *139:*690-719, 1954.

Sparkman, R. S., and Wu, S.: Subcapsular rupture of the liver following indefinite injury. J. A. M. A., *179:*226-228, 1962.

Spector, N.: Ligation of the right hepatic artery in hemobilia. Report of a case with recovery. Ann. Surg., *145:*244-248, 1957.

Still, E. U.: On the toxicity of purified bile preparations. Amer. J. Physiol., *88:*729-736, 1929.

Stone, F. A., et al.: Treatment of exsanguinating rupture of the right lobe of the liver by ligation of the main hepatic artery. Case report. Ann. Surg., *162:*933-937, 1965.

Thomas, C. S., Jr., Adkins, R. B., Jr., Lanier, V. C., Jr., and Foster, J. H.: The surgical management of intrahepatic hematomas. Amer. Surg., *36:*171-176, 1970.

Thors, R., Grindlay, J. H., and Bollman, J. L.: Effect of ligation of the hepatic artery on oxygen content of blood from the hepatic vein in dogs. Surg. Forum, *3:*500-504, 1952.

Tilton, B. T.: Some considerations regarding wounds of the liver. Ann. Surg., *41:*20-30, 1905.

Vasko, J. S., and Scott, H. W., Jr.: Acute renal failure from massive intrahepatic hematoma compressing the inferior vena cava: recovery after right hepatic lobectomy. Ann. Surg., *163:*144-148, 1966.

Wangensteen, O. H.: On the significance of the escape of sterile bile into the peritoneal cavity. Ann. Surg., *84:*691-702, 1926.

Williams, L. F., Jr., and Byrne, J. J.: Trauma to the liver at Boston City Hospital from 1955 to 1965. Amer. J. Surg., *112:*368-375, 1966.

Index

Page numbers in *italics* indicate figures; page numbers followed by t indicate tables.